As my Body
Attacks Itself

As my Body Attacks Itself

My journey with autoimmune disease, chronic pain and fatigue

Kelly Morgan Dempewolf, PhD

First Printing, 2014

ISBN 978-0-9862971-0-6

K$_2$CS Books
Tecumseh, KS 66542

www.asmybodyattacksitself.com

Table of Contents

To Caleb & shana
because I wish I'd given you better genes!

Forward

More than 50 million people have been diagnosed with autoimmune disease. There are many stories illustrating how the diagnosis not only takes a physical toll on a patient but also affects them emotionally, psychologically and financially. Within these tales of extreme pain and uncertainty underlies one common theme: the amount of time that it takes to receive an accurate diagnosis.

A 2014 American Autoimmune Related Diseases Association (AARDA) survey revealed that it takes four years and five different physicians for a patient to receive an accurate diagnosis. As in Kelly's case, many patients are labeled chronic complainers and their concerns dismissed. If concerns are not dismissed, patients can be prescribed a variety of medications. Many times, without an exact diagnosis, these medications can potentially exacerbate a patient's condition.

Not only are bodies being drained physically but so are finances. AARDA has heard Kelly's concerns. In an effort to alleviate patient suffering, AARDA distributed a physician survey to gauge how much autoimmune disease education they received in medical school. The results are alarming. The survey showed that 13% of the respondents didn't receive any autoimmune disease education at all while only 22% received five or more lectures. Sadly, 32% believed that they didn't receive enough training to diagnose or treat autoimmune disease and half of those that responded were uncomfortable with diagnosing autoimmune disease.

These results are why Kelly's story is so timely and needed. Her chronicles are relatable and speak to the need of increased autoimmune disease education. Hopefully, readers will not overlook Kelly's bravery and only see only the challenges that she has endured. We hope that patients find strength to speak up and speak out about autoimmune disease. Writing letters to their Congressperson, participating in awareness walks and taking their stories to the local media are only a few ways to take action. Awareness and education depends on us...the 50 million with autoimmune disease.

Virginia T. Ladd
Executive Director and President of the American Autoimmune Related Diseases Association (AARDA)

Introduction

This book began as a blog. It was meant as a way for me to work through what had been going on the last few years. It was a way for me to communicate to my family and friends. My emotions always get in the way when I try to talk about it, but writing gives me enough distance that I can "get it out".

However, I quickly found an online community of autoimmune disease patients and began sharing my writings with them as I read through their blogs and tweets. That's when an amazing thing happened - people I'd never met or interacted with before began commenting on the blog and emailing me. They were reaching out to let me know that I was able to put into words what they were feeling. One even included my blog URL in the signature section of all the emails he sent in hopes that his friends and family would read it and gain a better understanding of what he was going through.

I was blown away by this - I never expected this kind of response from strangers! I began to realize that maybe my writing could provide a voice for others in addition to myself. Maybe it would help others uncover their own struggles, as it's often hard to pinpoint exactly what it is about this autoimmune disease journey that has you frustrated, angry, sad, scared, etc. It's often so overwhelming in the whole that it's hard to break it down into specifics, which I think is necessary if we want to work through and communicate our struggles.

That's when the blog became a book - something that could be read by other autoimmune patients to help them with their own journey and something they could share with those in their lives to help them understand what it's like to live with such insidious diseases.

Just like the signs and symptoms of various autoimmune diseases are often similar and over-lapping, the personal struggles the sufferers go through are similar as well. So although I'll talk briefly about my specific autoimmune disease condition, I truly think this book applies to all autoimmune conditions, and for that matter all invisible chronic diseases! This book is for anyone touched by chronic diseases - their own disease or that of a loved one or patient.

As you read this, please remember that my point of writing this is not to whine about what's going on with me, or to imply that what is going on with me is all-important and all others in my life should be constantly aware of it. It's to help me process my feelings and emotions, to give others insight into what it's like to live with these issues and to maybe help someone else dealing with similar things to process their own experiences.

This book is an honest, raw look at my thoughts, concerns, fears and struggles. It scares me immensely to admit many of the things that I talk about in this book - it's bad enough to have to admit them to myself, but to make them public in book form is terrifying. But it's also liberating and satisfying. If my writings can help others then maybe that will be the one bright side to this journey I'm stuck on - maybe that's the point behind it all for me.

My hope is that patients will find solace and validation; friends and family will gain understanding and the abilities to empathize, communicate and support loved ones; and medical professionals will gain understanding and ability to empathize - impacting the way they interact with patients.

I hurt

I hurt.

All the time.

Every day.

Since about January 2011.

I've experienced physical pain at various points in my life - I had shingles in 9th grade, two knee surgeries when I was 20 years old, a broken rib (while having to perform ballet on stage - pas de deux en pointe - and without screaming every time my partner picked me up or I took a deep breath, or frankly every time I moved for that matter). I gave birth to two children (not to mention was pregnant with each of them for 9 months before the birth and it felt like one of them was trying to pry my ribs apart with her little hands during the last couple of months). I've had back muscle spasms, cracked molars and a crown-lengthening (which I have to say was probably the worst acute pain I've experienced!)

Of course no history of my pain and/or injuries would be complete without mentioning that my brother cut part of my pinky off in a door when I was little. OK, so I don't really remember the pain from that experience because I was too young at the time, but I'm sure there had to be pain, right?! I mean getting the end of a finger cut off has GOT to painful! But, mostly, I just like bringing it up any chance I get over the last 30+ years because I know it irritates my big brother…and really, what other reason do you need when you have that one. You're welcome, Chris.

However, all of those instances were acute. They were temporary. I knew they would end and life would return to normal. That knowledge is more comforting than I, and I think most people, ever realized.

I now suffer from chronic illness. I have an autoimmune disease that, among other things, causes chronic pain and fatigue. My pain is usually in my hands, wrists and feet. It is a constant, aching, interfering-in-my-activities type of pain. Some days are better and some are worse, but it's always there.

I like to think of myself as a caring, empathetic, and sympathetic person. However I truly had no idea of the ramifications chronic pain has in the lives of those that suffer from it until I began experiencing it for myself.

I think I could imagine the physical pain piece of chronic pain. But the toll it would take on my relationships and self-concept, as well as on my mental and emotional health, was not something I could have imagined until I experienced it. I could have envisioned chronic pain impacting mental and emotional health, but I couldn't have begun to imagine just exactly what that would be like.

I'm sorry if this sounds rude or somehow self-righteous or elitist (believe me I'd rather not be in this group even if it were "elite") - but I don't think anyone truly understands what it's like until they've lived it.

I don't share most of the things that go through my mind and emotions I feel, because I don't think others would be interested; because everyone has their own problems and they don't need mine; because I don't want to wear out my welcome; because I truly think they don't understand until they've experienced it; and because I'm ashamed of how I feel. And, increasingly so, because I'm just tired. I'm worn out from all of this and just don't feel like talking about it.

So why am I writing about it now? Well, for one, because my therapist encouraged me. I began meeting with her when I was going through a divorce. Several years after that I'm still seeing her, because, frankly, I think the world would be a better place if we all had one.

Over the years she's seen my passion for education. I was a high school chemistry teacher for 10 years and I still work in education. But I'm not just an educator; I'm someone that wants to continually work towards changing things for the better. I'm active in the dialogue on changing/improving education and believe passionately in my two "causes" - (1) encouraging and supporting as many teachers as possible to transition to student-paced mastery learning in their classrooms and (2) helping teachers develop the scientist in every student through authentic scientific processes. I write and speak about those topics and truly believe they can change the way our children are educated for the better.

So what does that have to do with me writing about my pain and health issues? I'm a pretty verbal person - I write. If writing about my experiences, thoughts and feelings could help me work through what I'm going through then that's got to be a good thing. If finding my voice helps me to advocate for myself and seek what I need to move forward then that's also a good thing. If sharing that writing with others could help someone else process what they're going through, or help a loved one, caregiver or medical professionals see what it's like to live with chronic illness, then...bonus!

I'm Tired

I'm tired.

Not every day, but more often than not.

Since at least 2007.

Just as I've experienced other types of pain, I've also experienced other types of exhaustion. I've stayed up too late, woken up too early, been physically drained by long days of dance, fatigued while healing from surgery, experienced restless nights during pregnancy and had many, many nights awake with each of my kids when they were babies.

I first talked to my doctor about fatigue at my annual appointment in early 2008. At that time, my kids were 2 & 4 years old, I was teaching high school science and I was still married to my ex-husband. I would push through work during the week and taking care of the kids each night and I'd get to the weekends and my body would give out. I'd lay down on the couch, fall asleep, and not be able to drag myself out of it. And this was with regular, solid sleep of 8 hours or more each night.

No amount of "catching up" or "extra sleep" made it go away. I knew something wasn't right with me. I knew this was more than "you have 2 little kids and work hard" tired. This was deep-down fatigue. The closest I can come to explaining it is the fatigue women experience during the first trimester of pregnancy - but even that isn't quite exactly what it's like. I've also heard it described as being like having the flu continuously for years - with varying intensity. It's not always at it's worst, but it is always there.

Everyone has been tired. Everyone has felt so exhausted that they can't do a single thing more. Imagine being that exhausted - as physically and mentally drained as you've ever been - on a regular basis. And with no justifiable reason. It's one thing to be exhausted when you have a reason - when you can explain it. But it's another to know that you should not be feeling this way based on your recent sleep and activity level.

And as if it's not bad enough to be experiencing something that you know you have no good reason to be experiencing, having others see it (and judge it) is a million times worse. It took three years from the first time I went to the doctor for fatigue to receive a diagnosis (more about that later). During those three years I had "no good reason" for feeling the way that I was feeling. For the first of those three years I was still married to my ex-husband. Not only did I not understand what was going on with me, he certainly did not and he didn't even have the advantage I had of physically feeling it for himself. I was called lazy, made to feel guilty and accused of making it all up (especially after I came back from the specialist my primary care doctor sent me to see in 2008 without a diagnosis that explained it). I had nothing to point to be able to explain, describe or justify it. In fact, I had a doctor that said I didn't have a medical reason - so not only could I not justify it, I had a medical *professional* that said there was no reason for it.

It's easier now that I have a diagnosis - it's easier to explain to others that I'm fatigued because of my disease. But they still can't see it and it still sounds like just an excuse. Everyone is tired. Everyone is busy. Why do I get to take a nap because I'm "fatigued"? Why do I not have to do as much around the house as my husband? Why do I say "no" to volunteering for things my kids are involved in or events at their school?

I'm sure that others think "yeah, right, fatigue" when I try to explain it. I'm sure they think "everyone is tired, why is hers so different?" I'm sure some think I'm lazy, not pulling my weight or not being the best parent, friend, etc.

Why do I think others are thinking these things? Because I'm thinking them about myself. Am I really sure that it's fatigue or am I being lazy? On the days when I feel better, it's tempting to say that it's in my head or that I'm exaggerating it. But then the days that are worse come again and I know there's no exaggeration. I would love to be my active, involved, efficient self again. I would not choose this fatigued life even if it did mean getting out of chores. It's just not worth it.

One of the frustrating things about this type of fatigue is that rest doesn't make it better. When you're tired because you haven't had enough sleep you can "catch up" on sleep and feel better. But no matter how many days include a nap and no matter how many nights I get 9+ hours of sleep, I still have the fatigue.

There are ways to cope with fatigue. For example, I'm learning to say no. I'm still not very good at it and still say yes sometimes when I shouldn't, but I am getting better. I realize that each time I say yes to something that I'm giving away a piece of my time, which I have even less of than most people because chunks of time are already taken out for fatigue. I've cut out many hobbies, reduced how much help out with the kids' activities and other things in my life - but I definitely still feel pressure to get various things done or be a part of different happenings.

I'm learning to prioritize, but there are so many things that aren't getting done - things that are being put off or skipped altogether. On the days where I do have more energy, it's hard to choose what to do. Should I take care of the lower priority things that have been being pushed from day to day on my to-do list because they don't get done when my energy levels are lower? Do I take that extra energy and time to enjoy something - like doing something fun with my kids - since so much of my available time is spent on tasks I have to do? Do I try to work towards long-term goals that I'm still holding on to, instead of getting lost in the minutia of the prioritized list of to-do's while I have a brief window of "energy"?

I'm learning to schedule an appropriate number of things for each day - but it's hard when you don't know if that day is going to be a high fatigue day or a day with more energy. It's like trying to create a shopping list when you're not sure how much money you're going to have that day. Then you get to the store and realize you have less than you thought - what do you cut out? Or what if you get there and realize you have more than you'd planned for - do you stock up on things for another time when you don't have as much? (This is where the money analogy breaks down - you can't store up extra energy like you can save extra money in a bank for another time!)

How do I explain and justify fatigue - to myself and others - when it just sounds like such an excuse?

Invisible Diseases

The invisible nature of these diseases is so different from "normal" illnesses and injuries that I have read often about people having to carefully construct their image when going into a doctor's appointment (particular if it's a new doctor). If you look too well put together they don't think you're really sick and hurting. If you look on the outside like you feel on the inside then they write you off as depressed and fail to take you seriously. There's an art to looking "credibly sick". It's ridiculous that this ever happens, but it most definitely does – many, many chronically ill have talked about it in blogs and on social media.

I talked about my various painful experiences a few chapters ago. They include the usual things people experience - injuries, surgeries and so forth. All acute (short-term), all things that would heal and my life would go on with the experience leaving behind nothing more than a memory and maybe a scar. However, chronic disease is forever. There is no cure.

Another difference between all of those painful experiences and my current painful autoimmune disease is that those were visible. Finger cut off: cast. Knee surgeries: knee brace. Thyroid surgery: healing line across my neck that looked like someone had tried to slit my throat. Pregnancy and child birth: I was visibly pregnant and then I had a newborn. With the exception of the rib fracture and tooth pain, there was always some visible sign as to what I was going through.

I don't want to be the center of attention. I know that everyone has their own lives and own issues. But the problem is that not only am I not the center of attention for my painful experiences (which I truly don't want), but it's very, very easy for people to forget. There's got to be a middle ground between "center of attention" and "everyone forgets."

And everyone forgetting in itself is not the issue. I don't need everyone to be constantly conscious of my pain level. But there are times when it would be helpful if I had an outward signal to show how I was feeling and that I had a valid reason to act the way I am.

For example, I was in college when I had my knee surgeries. My first knee surgery was right after my sophomore year ended and I had just moved into an apartment with a roommate for the summer. My parents had come out to help me move, and to be with me during my surgery, but after about a week they went back home. After they'd left, I was sitting on the couch in the living room with my leg up on the coffee table but I had my knee brace off. The phone rang (a real, honest-to-goodness house phone, we didn't have cell phones yet!) and I called out to my roommate to see if she could come answer it. She came in with a look on her face and said "Why can't you get it?" Then she looked at my leg on the coffee table, complete with swelling, stitches and bandages, and said "Oh, I'm sorry...I forgot! Of course!"

We tend to cut people slack when we are aware of their pain or discomfort. And an outward signal of that pain and discomfort helps us remember when we get busy with what's going on with ourselves and forget - which is completely normal and natural and I would never blame anyone for it.

I don't want slack for everything. I need and want to continue to live my life, to be a mother and wife, to continue to work. But I would like appropriate empathy and consideration when something is more difficult than it should be for me or when I'm a little crankier than usual because the pain is worse today.

My chronic pain has no outward sign. No one would look at my hands and realize the pain that I'm in. There's nothing visibly wrong with them. No one can look at them and see when it's a bad day (right now there are no "good days" - just "bad" and "not-so-bad"). If I'm not wanting to cook because holding the spoons and stirring hurts, or if I don't want to do laundry because grabbing the wet, tangled clothes out of the washer and putting them in the dryer is way more painful than doing laundry should be, it's easy for people to forget that there's a reason that I'm not doing those things. There's a reason that I'm not "doing my part"...because it literally *hurts*.

I don't want or expect everyone to constantly be aware of my pain level. And I don't want or expect to be given a free pass on everything - I can do some things and I want to do what I can for my family and friends. Also, I know that it's probably pretty vain of me, but on some level I'm glad I'm not visible injured - I don't want my hands to look disfigured or obviously wounded. But then again, it would be a lot easier to explain why I act the way I sometimes do if my disease wasn't invisible.

I went to an annual appointment with an optometrist in the fall of 2014 for a glasses prescription update. When I told him about my Sjögren's and the punctal plug process I'd been through that summer he was asking how bad my eye dryness was in my opinion – how much it affected my life. I answered his question, but then also included that compared to the fatigue and pain it's not even my most pressing concern, no matter how bad it is (and it is bad enough to be intrusive in my daily life). He was very surprised and said "well I wouldn't know to look at you – you look just fine." Hello. This doctor is working in one of the areas that deals with my disease. He acted as if he was familiar with it when I mentioned it during one of my son's previous appointments with him (during idol conversation about contacts and glasses). And here he was, a medical professional that is self-professed to be familiar with this disease and he says he wouldn't know by looking at me that I struggle with this disease. It's an INVISIBLE DISEASE – there's nothing that would show you outwardly that I was having these problems. If medical professionals working in a specialty area that deals with the disease have this kind of obvious misconception about the invisible nature of it, it's no wonder that everyone else does as well!

Degenerative Diseases

There's a special kind of torture with being diagnosed with a degenerative disease. Added on to the chronic pain, chronic fatigue and struggles with dealing with an invisible disease, there's something just that much worse about degenerative diseases.

For a while my primary diagnosis was Rheumatoid Arthritis. (More about my current diagnosis later!) RA can get very bad, very quickly or it can be relatively stable for quite a while.

I was diagnosed with it before my husband and I were married. I was extremely serious when I let him know that I would understand if he didn't want to marry me after finding this out. This can be a debilitating disease that could cause me to lose the ability to use my hands. I could lose the ability to dress myself or take care of myself in even the most basic of ways.

Yes, it is true that *no one* knows what the future may hold for them. They may be in a car accident, be diagnosed with cancer or have a million other tragic things happen in their lifetime. But the difference between those "what-ifs" and the "what-ifs" after you're diagnosed with a degenerative disease is an important one.

No one knows what may happen to them in their life-time, but when you're diagnosed with a life-long degenerative disease, you know *something* is going to happen. You don't know when and you don't know how bad it will be, but you know it's coming. You know that it will take away even more from your life than it's already taken. You know that it will cause you to rely on those around you - that you may become a burden much earlier than you ever expected.

On the one hand, it causes you to appreciate the days that you do have before it worsens. You learn to appreciate the things that you can still do for yourself. You have the feeling of wanting to live your life to fullest while you can.

Except that you can't.

You're still battling chronic pain and fatigue. You're still going from one medication to another, trying to find one that will work. It's not a matter of "I'm fine now but I know something bad will happen to me later, so I'll live it up now." Instead, it's "I'm not fine now, in fact I'm so bad that I finally have gone to doctors seeking help and I can't live my life as normal - let alone live it up - and I know that at some point it's going to get even worse than it is now."

And some autoimmune diseases make it just about impossible to forget that it is a degenerative process. The pain that is associated with RA is due to inflammation in the joints. Not only does this inflammation cause pain, it does damage. And it's permanent damage. The longer that the inflammation goes uncontrolled the more damage is happening. Therefore the pain is a constant reminder that your body is getting worse right at that very moment. You have this reminder that this pain isn't just pain and it's not just something you can tough through or cover up with pain medication. As long as the pain is there, you know the inflammation is there. As long as the inflammation is there, you know it's causing more damage.

So, yes, no one knows what tragic and life-altering circumstances may happen in their future. However, they do not know for a *certainty* that something will happen. They also do not have a constant reminder that it *will* happen. These are issues that people with degenerative diseases do have.

How would you rate your pain today?

Each time I go a doctor, even if it is unrelated to the conditions that are causing me pain, I'm asked "do you have any pain today?"

I often chuckle at this question. I know they're well-meaning, and I'm not laughing at the nurse. My chuckle is more of a shaking-my-head-in-resignation reflex. Because I'm always in pain. It's similar to the "does a bear..." question.

I answer "yes" and then am asked "How long have you had it?"

This question again makes me laugh to myself, this time at what has become a massive amount of time with no comfort, as I answer "um, coming up on four years."

The third question in this series is "On a scale of 1 to 10, with 10 being the worst pain you could ever imagine, what would you rate your pain?"

This is the question that always gets me. "The worst pain you could ever imagine." As soon as they say that phrase I immediately down-grade the number I probably would have given had that phrase not been included in the question. It instantly makes me think "surely this is nowhere near the worst pain I could imagine." I think there's a couple reason for this pain-scale-downgrade process.

First of all, I am fully aware that there are always people in the world worse off than I am. I don't want to seem ungrateful, I don't want to seem like I'm saying I'm as bad as the people dealing with things far worse. Even if that thought never crosses the nurse's mind, I don't want to seem to *myself* (in my own mind) that I'm equating my issues with those that are struggling with more. Intellectually I know that this is a ridiculous reason to downgrade my pain scale rating, but it's the reality of what's happening with me.

Second, some days are better than others. The pain is never gone, but some days are better than others. If I rate my current pain as higher on the scale and then days, weeks, or months later it gets worse than I imagined it would…I'll have no place to go on the scale. If I "top out" or "overrate" then how will I communicate when it's getting even worse?

Then there's the issue of for what time period I'm supposed to report a rating. Do I give a rating for only that moment - an instant pain rating. Or an average for the day as a whole? Or what about an average since the last time I've been to the doctor? Sometimes an instantaneous pain rating isn't indicative of my overall pain level. I want to make sure that what I'm giving a rating for is the same as how the health professional is interpreting it so that we're communicating effectively.

So I go through the process of thinking to myself "what's a reasonable number for my issues?" What's a reasonable number for pain in my hands, wrists and feet compared to someone that was crushed in a car accident or burned over most of their body (apparently, those are the types of pain that would be the worst I could imagine)? Surely those must be "10" type pains. And if that's what a 10 is then mine must be only a 3! After all, there's a big difference between my situation and those!

But if I rate it too low will the doctors take it seriously? Will they realize that I am truly in constant pain and work to understand or relieve it?

So then I do the strange thing of giving a range: "3 to 4, I guess." Really? I can't just pick a number? And why do I always add "I guess"? I'm a mess!

Then, as if this simple process of rating my pain on a scale of 1-10 couldn't get any more unnecessarily complicated, sometimes the office will have a poster that not only contains the 1-10 scale with the smiley faces, but they also have descriptors about how the pain is affecting your day.

On these posters, the phrase "can be ignored" appears under the "1-3" range. Well, mine definitely cannot be ignored.

So then I look at the next range "interferes with tasks" is shown under the "3-5" range. My pain definitely interferes with tasks (not to mention my mood). OK, so maybe that's a better place for me - but I'd better check the next level up to see if I fit in that one.

"Interferes with concentration" is below the "5-7" range. Oh. Well, yeah, my pain does that. Maybe I should rate it higher. I'd better check the next level…

"Interferes with basic needs" and "bed rest required" are the top two categories. OK, I'm not there yet.

Going by these descriptions, it seems that most of the time I'm in the "5-7" range. But I bet if I went through the medical records of all my various appointments, "3" is probably my most common response. So why do I have such a hard time expressing a number in the "5-7" range to my doctors? Does everyone have this issue?

My 9 year-old daughter certainly doesn't seem to have these issues - she has no problem pointing to the dark red frowny face under the number 6 or even the orange deeper-frowny-face under the 8 when she has a sore throat or pink eye. Why is she so able to express how she really feels while I am not? Is it my age/experience along with the realization that there are much worse things in the world going on than what I'm dealing with? Or is it something about me, my personality or the way I think?

Or is it because her pain and discomfort is acute - it wasn't there the day (or couple of days) before and it won't be there (hopefully) within a day or two after. She knows what she feels like when she's feeling good and she knows how she feels right at that moment isn't good. She can easily compare the "before" with the "after." She knows how she's feeling now isn't normal.

I've been in daily pain since January 2011. Unfortunately this has become my "new normal." I truly don't remember what it is like to not have pain. I have some vague understanding of "it's better than this," but beyond that I really don't know. Has the chronic nature of my discomfort somehow shifted my ability to communicate to others the severity of my pain? And if so, how can I more effectively communicate it to the nurses and doctors?

Beyond a Pain Scale

The more pro-active I become in my disease diagnosis and management, the more time I spend thinking about exactly how to phrase things and exactly how to communicate to medical professionals.

My symptoms are often difficult to describe as they are not typical things such as pain that we all have words to describe. For example, the best way I could describe my fine motor controls issues for a while was to say "my hands don't do what my brain tells them." When that description didn't lead to a doctor's understanding, or being able to describe it accurately in his or her dictation, or being able to figure out the correct tests and diagnostic tools, I spent a lot of time thinking about how to describe it better. I spent time doing nothing other than analyzing what exactly is going on when a symptom is especially intrusive in my life during a given moment. Is it numbness? No. Is it tingling? No. Is it weakness? Yes, that's part of it. Is it pain? Not exactly. What motions are difficult? Bending fingers down - such as to wave, type, squeeze, hold a pencil, etc. Does it feel tight when I do it? No, not really. It's more that it feels slow - it take a more deliberate movement to make it happen correctly. Where do you feel it? Back of the hand.

And that's just how I sit and analyzed one symptom one

time it showed itself. There's also the fatigue, the weakness, the brain fog and all the other things that I'll talk about in this book. These things all affect my life. They all make it difficult to think, work, do my personal and home activities and in general just be myself.

So when a nurse or doctor simply asks about my pain rating on a scale of 1 to 10, that's just the tip of the iceberg. In fact, sometimes my pain is the least of the factors interfering with my ability to function normally. I believe that a much better question to ask would be "how able are you to function through your normal daily tasks on a scale of 1 to 10 with 1 being 'without interference from my disease', and 10 being 'I cannot complete any work, family, social, personal or other daily tasks due to my disease.'"

The follow-up question (like the "where is your pain?" "what kind of pain?" and "how long have you had it?" that always come after the pain scale question) can be "what things are causing this change in your ability to complete normal daily tasks?" to which the patient can list the symptoms currently causing them problems such as fatigue, muscle weakness, dry eyes, etc. They can ask "how long can you ignore these symptoms if doing something very important?" There are times that I can push through and complete something that has got to be done (especially when it involves taking care of my kids) but how long I'm able to keep pushing and ignore the symptoms is an indication of how bad they are at that moment.

There's so much more to this than pain and I think using that as the only metric by which we gauge disease activity or patient discomfort is a grave injustice.

So what exactly do you have?

I'm often asked "So what exactly do you have?" That's a good question! It took me five years to figure it out! And I'm not totally convinced that the story is complete yet.

There are over 80 autoimmune diseases. And we know so very little known about them! They're complex, can involve every organ in the body and their signs and symptoms can mimic each other and so many other diseases that diagnosing them sometimes feels like throwing a dart at a dartboard.

The various autoimmune diseases can all have similar lab work and symptoms. Fatigue, joint pain, and blood work with high rheumatoid factor and sed rate (a test for inflammation in the body) could be present in probably every single one of those 80+ autoimmune diseases.

And to make it worse, sometimes they can't identify what you have exactly. You have bits and pieces of various ones and they diagnose you with "Undifferentiated Connective Tissue Disease." I'm pretty sure that's just a catch-all diagnosis when they can't figure out exactly what you have, or maybe they haven't "named" the specific disease you have yet - it hasn't been differentiated from the many other autoimmune diseases. It's hard enough to explain to others what's going on with you when you have a definite diagnosis (that they've likely never heard of before) - try explaining that you have a vague conglomerate of many things but yet none of them individually!

My only currently confirmed diagnosis is Sjögren's Syndrome (pronounced SHOW-grins). I know…you're thinking "What is that? I've never heard of that!" Most people haven't.

Our immune systems are what keep us healthy - they attack things in the body that aren't supposed to be there and that may be trying to do us harm (such as germs). However in some people (and they have no clear idea why or how), the immune system begins to attack things that *should* be there and not only are those things not trying to harm us, but they are actually *necessary* to our well-being! (Hence the name of this book "As my body attacks itself.")

Approximately 4 million Americans are living with Sjögren's today. That's about 1.3% of the country's population, or about 1 out of every 100 people. Nine out of ten of the people with Sjögren's are women. Yay, us!

There seems to be a "sweet spot" with respect to age for diagnosis and for people reacting to what's going on with you in a way that reaffirms what's happening.

I was 31 when I first reported symptoms to my PCP and optometrist. I know that I was younger than that when symptoms first began showing up. It took a while for the "symptom creep" to get to the point that I began discussing it with my doctors. Likely, it was my mid to late 20's when it started.

The information on Sjögren's says that symptoms typically begin between ages 45 and 55, although I doubt that being in that "sweet spot" means diagnosis happens much more quickly. It still takes putting together seemingly desperate symptoms into one diagnosis and that will likely take a long time and many doctors visits before it happens, no matter your age.

However when you're younger than the "sweet spot" people tend to tell you that you're too young and write it off. The symptoms must be a fluke, or in your head, or not as big of a deal as you're making them.

I imagine that when you're older than the "sweet spot" people write it off as aging. Dry eyes and mouth, as well as joint pain and brain fog (all symptoms of Sjögren's), naturally increase as a person ages. But this disease goes beyond appropriate symptoms for the aging process - it's pronounced symptoms.

It seems all too easy to look at "average" and "typical" and forget that there are outliers in every "average." It's already too easy to ignore symptoms of these diseases - simple because of the invisible and "creeping" nature of them - age doesn't need to be yet another reason to ignore them.

Autoimmune diseases are differentiated by what exactly they attack in our body. Sjögren's is when the white-blood cells in the body attack the moisture-producing glands, such as those producing saliva and tears.

So at this point you're probably thinking something along the lines of "so just use eye drops and drink water to replace the tears and saliva you're missing." That's what I thought, too. I first heard about this disease and wrote it off as something "minor" compared to whatever else had to be causing all of these other problems in my body.

I wasn't diagnosed with Sjögren's until almost 5 years after my first report of symptoms to a doctor. And it came 2 years after the incorrect diagnosis of Rheumatoid Arthritis. So when my doctor added in this diagnosis, I thought "Big deal - low tears and spit. That's minor compared to the pain and possible damage to my body due to more serious diseases that are happening."

At least that's how I thought about it until I found out all the other lovely things about Sjögren's syndrome.

Sjögren's can also affect the kidneys, gastrointestinal system, blood vessels, lungs, liver, pancreas and central nervous system. Sjögren's is systemic - it affects the entire body! Sjögren's patients also have an increased rate of lymphoma. Ummm…OK, so this is more serious than "just throw in some artificial tears and drink some water when you eat."

Symptoms include, along with the dry eyes, mouth, nose, skin and vagina, "extreme fatigue and joint pain."* The symptoms can remain constant, get worse or go into remission (although that's rare…dang it!) People experience it differently - from mild discomfort to debilitating symptoms.

The problem is, like I mentioned before, autoimmune diseases mimic each other. That, combined with the fact that not only is the general public awareness for this disease extremely low (especially when you consider the prevalence of the disease), but even medical professional awareness is not where it should be. Therefore, it takes an average of 4.7 years to receive a diagnosis of Sjögren's. And that's just about how long it took me to receive my diagnosis. (Although the wonderful

---

*   www.sjogrens.org

Sjögren's Syndrome Foundation, www.Sjögrens.org, is working very, very hard to decrease the time of diagnosis by half in 5 years through education efforts and they're making progress, but even an average diagnosis time of 2.5 years, their goal, is far too long in my opinion!)

There are two antibodies that can show up in blood work (SS-A and SS-B) that are fairly specific for Sjögren's (SS-B is even more specific than SS-A). However I wasn't even tested for those antibodies until the doctor suspected the disease, almost 5 years in. And that only happened when I switched doctors - who knows if or when my original rheumatologist would have tested me…or even proposed the idea that I might have this disease! Turns out, I have both antibodies.

It can also be diagnosed with a variety of tests on the eyes to see how dry they are and how you produce tears. I pretty much flunked those tests…and in fact flunked so poorly that I was told I couldn't wear contacts…forever. Lip biopsies are also a diagnostic tool – I've been spared that because I had the antibodies and dry eye tests confirm the diagnosis already.

Disease Envy

There are many times throughout the last few years of dealing with this chronic illness that I've been unable to express what I'm feeling and thinking. There are many reasons for it - fear of how others will look at me, not wanting to be the "girl who cried pain" or appearing narcissistic. But on the topic of disease envy, the things that keep my from expressing my feelings are not wanting to appear insensitive to other's health struggles or offending them, and frankly, not wanting to sound stupid.

But here goes. Yes, I envy other diseases.

I do not want other diseases - I wish no one had them. I do not want this to seem insensitive or flippant in any way. I do not think my disease is worse than others. It's just that I envy things about other diseases. If I have to have a disease, there are aspects of others that I would prefer.

It's hard having something that takes an average of almost 5 years to be diagnosed. It's hard having something that no one has heard of. It's hard having something that people write off as being a "nuisance" rather than something serious. It's hard having something that doesn't get much attention in the general public, that has no "awareness" presence.

Diabetes is straight-forward to diagnose and treat. Not that there aren't terrible long-term problems with diabetes. One of my dear friends that I've known since junior high has Type I diabetes (which actually is an autoimmune disease as well). It's severe and we've talked about the mental challenges with having something that you know can lead to degenerative problems over the years. She's also a vet and even she admits she'd rather treat animals with diabetes than other autoimmune disorders. Diabetes is by no means easy, but it is easy to diagnose and treat. People know what it is. There's awareness and understanding. There's research going on and medical professionals know to look for it when people come in with relevant symptoms.

My paternal grandmother and paternal aunt had breast cancer. My aunt died from it. I began having mammograms earlier than the usual age of 40 because of this family history. I hope to God that I never have to deal with it. I pray that my daughter never has to deal with it. I wish no one did. But it is on everyone's radar. Medical professions are well-aware of the importance of early detection. Breast exams are a part of annual physicals, they always instruct the patients on doing them in between physicals and mammograms are routine testing for women at higher risk. The public is very aware. The awareness for breast cancer is so large that it has made its way into NASCAR, the NFL, yogurt containers and just about everything else. Yes, breast cancer is life-threatening and for people, like my aunt, it can be life-ending, and that's horrible. Complications from Sjögren's (lung and kidney complications or the greater chance of lymphoma) can be as well. Autoimmune diseases as a group are listed in the top 10 causes of death and the 4th leading cause of disability for women.

Again, I'm not saying that my disease is worse. I'm not saying I'd rather have these other diseases or issues. I wish no one had any of them. But there are aspects of the other disease that I envy, like the ability to be definitively diagnosed with a lab test or biopsy instead of a pool of vague and often non-present symptoms or blood markers (some of which may only work for about half of the people with a given autoimmune disease).

The awareness, support and research - both in the general public and the medical community - is also something I envy a great deal. People immediately know what these other diseases are and immediately realize they're serious. Medical professional are acutely aware of them and understand the importance of early diagnosis and quick treatment.

I know that people can't know about every disease under the moon - we can't all be experts in every disease that those around us may or may not have. But approximately 50 million Americans have an auto-immune disease[*]. That's 16 out of every 100 people. Approximately 4 million Americans have Sjögren's Syndrome (1 out of every 100 people).

Here are some facts comparing autoimmune disease with cancer. Again - not saying one is worse than the other, just trying to compare autoimmune disease numbers with something with which people are more familiar.

---

[*]   American Autoimmune Related Disease Association (http://www.aarda.org/autoimmune-information/autoimmune-statistics/)

	Autoimmune disease (not including Type 1 Diabetes)	Cancer
Number of Americans	47 million	11 million
Research funding (2013)	$821 million	$5.3 billion

2013 funding figures from NIH[†]

Type 1 diabetes ("juvenile diabetes") is an autoimmune disease but has been excluded from these numbers as it is difficult to separate the funding spent on Type 1 diabetes from that spent on Type 2 diabetes (which is not an autoimmune disease).

There are 4 times as many people with autoimmune disease in this country as cancer. To put the research funding in a per-person perspective, there is $17.47 for each person with autoimmune disease and $481.82 for each person with cancer. I'm not saying everything has to be even - and I most definitely want cancer research to continue and be effective - but with autoimmune disease affecting so many people in this country, can't the public awareness and research support increase even a little?

[†]   National Institute of Health (http://report.nih.gov/categorical_spending.aspx#legend5)

The Road to Diagnosis

It's been a very long, and meandering, path to diagnosis…and it still may not be over. Although I have one firm diagnosis (Sjögren's syndrome), people with one autoimmune disease are more likely to develop a second. And there's always the possibility that I have more than one now and that the second one hasn't been diagnosed or is being covered up by the first.

These diseases are masters of trickery. They act like each other. Symptoms come and go. They creep up without someone realizing just how bad they're getting. They overlap. Each person may have a unique presentation and history of the disease. No wonder they're so hard to diagnose!

I went to my primary care physician in early 2008 for the fatigue that I was experiencing. My PCP listened, as I feel like she always did and ran some blood work. She found elevated protein levels and sent me to a rheumatologist, we'll call her "Dr. A". I was nervous - as I always get when I need to see a specialist. I would guess most people feel that way.

In March of 2008, Dr. A gave me what I felt like (at the time) was a thorough exam. She told me nothing was wrong with me and it was probably just "life stress" that was causing my fatigue. I knew it was more than that, but I tend (like I think most people do) to try to take what a doctor says as correct. So I went on my way, knowing that the fatigue I felt wasn't right, but with nothing to point to that would explain it, I went on.

Fast forward 3 years - to spring of 2011. Lots had changed in my life - divorce, new house, new job, I was engaged to a wonderful man. Yet the fatigue had never really left - I would go through periods of time that were better than others, but it was never really gone.

And now I was having heart palpitations. Often. Enough to freak me out - especially considering that I knew two people my age that had died of heart attacks in the previous two years.

I went to the walk-in health clinic one night because I was worried enough to not wait until my own doctor's office opened. The doctor there listened to my heart, asked about my symptoms and felt like it wasn't really anything going on with my heart. She suggested it might be thyroid related and had my blood drawn. When she brought that up, I remembered that at my annual exam the previous year my PCP had noted that my thyroid felt large and was going to refer me for a sonogram. But somewhere along the line that referral got lost - the office referral department never called me with an appointment and I had forgotten about it. That is, until this walk-in clinic doctor mentioned that my palpitations may be caused by thyroid problems. She said she was going to refer me for a sonogram as well.

That referral office never called back, either.

About a week or so later, the palpitations where so

concerning and consistent that I went to the ER at night. They hooked me up, monitored my heart, took a bunch of blood and pulled up the results of the thyroid tests the walk-in doctor had ordered for me the week before. They said the thyroid tests were fine. They said they could see the palpitations that I was having on the monitor but they weren't the kind that causes them to worry, that some people have them their entire life. What did cause worry, though, was why I had started having them all of the sudden and so frequently. So I was sent home with instructions to make an appointment with my PCP.

My PCP began several rounds of blood work - each time she'd find something unusual and she'd order a more specific test. I felt like a pin cushion! She had me wear a heart monitor for a few days. And I finally got scheduled for that thyroid sonogram.

Turns out I had a nodule on my thyroid - and even though my thyroid labs were always normal, it was large enough that the surgeon felt it should come out. They took it out and the heart palpitations stopped that day. I haven't had them since. Yay, problem solved!

Only the real problems were just beginning. In the process of pulling all the blood work to solve the mystery of my heart palpitations, my PCP found that my sed rate was high - that's a measure of inflammation in the body but it's very non-specific. Lots of things can cause that. So then she drew blood to test a variety of things that could be causing it. She found my rheumatoid factor was high.

My doctor called. Herself. After office hours. When I answered the phone I knew that couldn't be good. Usually nurses call you - and even then they only call if things aren't good. I'd experienced that three days earlier when the nurse called me 15 minutes after I'd left the thyroid sonogram even though the technician had told me it would take several days for them to read the sonogram and get back to me...I knew that wasn't good either! When things are normal they just send a letter.

She told me my rheumatoid factor was very high and said "You have rheumatoid arthritis." She said she was setting up a referral to a rheumatologist. The rheumatoid arthritis had nothing to do with my heart palpitations (those were caused by the thyroid nodule, as evidenced by the fact that they completely stopped when my thyroid was removed) - it just happened to be found because of the searching we were doing for the cause of the heart palpitations. She had followed blood work down another path and discovered this as well. Had this not happened, I would have continued to explain away and fail to connect my various autoimmune symptoms (which right around that time started to include the joint pain, but I was so preoccupied with the heart palpitations that I didn't think much about it).

For years I believed this to be true - that the thyroid nodule and my autoimmune disease were two separate issues. However, now that I know I have Sjögren's and have learned more about the manifestations of the disease, thyroid nodules are fairly common in Sjögren's patients. There's no way to know for certain what caused my thyroid nodule - whether it was some random process in my body or if it was related to the Sjögren's. But I'm no longer certain that the two things are completely unrelated as I was in 2011.

A couple of days after her phone call to let me know about the RA diagnosis, I thought "hey, didn't I go see a rheumatologist a few years ago?" I called my PCP's nurse to ask if she could copy any information about that visit for me. She copied the letter that was sent from the rheumatologist ("Dr. A") to my PCP after my visit in March 2008.

The first page and a 3/4 described my history and the examination. The beginning stated that she was aware that the original concern was fatigue and that I was referred to her office because of the fatigue and blood work that showed elevated proteins. I read through it thinking not much was going to help me...I already knew all of the things she was saying.

Then, there it was in the last paragraph. A few sentences that reading now feels like someone has punched me in the gut.

In March 2008 she wrote:
> "Polyclonal gammopathies [the type of proteins I had that were elevated - the reason I'd been sent there] are usually seen in either infections or autoimmune inflammatory diseases. This patient doesn't give a history that is very suggestive of infection and there are no clues on examination to know where to start looking for one. Likewise, she does not have historical or physical findings of any of the usual rheumatologic autoimmune disorders."

But I *did* have two physical symptoms - extreme fatigue and these elevated proteins. I felt like if I'd pushed harder in 2008 maybe I'd have had a three year head-start compared to just starting the journey to diagnosis in 2011.

And now that I know even more about what I have, Sjögren's syndrome, I'm even crankier when I re-read this paragraph in the letter from 2008. Because although I didn't put it together in 2008, or even 2011, I've now figured out that I not only had *two* physical symptoms but that I had *four*, even back in 2008!

See, 2008 was also the year I began complaining to my optometrist that my eyes were so dry that my contacts were uncomfortable. She changed brands and was sure that would fix it - I even remember the phrase she used: "These are so comfortable that you'll think I'm a goddess for how great you feel." The new lenses only barely made it more comfortable, but I didn't push it any farther…after all, these were the newest, latest, greatest contacts on the market. Clearly I should be feeling great in them, so if I'm not, I'll just keep my mouth shut. I know. That's completely messed up. But somehow the fact that I should feel great in them kept me from speaking up that I *didn't* feel great in them.

I also know that I had dry mouth in 2008, too - it's been many years since I'd been able to take a bite of food and swallow it without taking a drink along with each bite.

There's no way I could have put together the symptoms of fatigue, dry eyes, dry mouth and elevated proteins and known they were all symptoms of the same systemic disease. How would I have ever known to associate those things together - they seemed so unrelated.

At first I think "well, then why does it upset you that Dr. A didn't put it together in 2008 either?" And for that matter, Dr. A never put it together - it was when I switched to Dr. B in March 2013 (5 years after my initial encounter with Dr. A) that I was first asked if I had dry eyes and dry mouth.

It upsets me because Sjögren's syndrome is the second

most common autoimmune disorder. And rheumatologists are exactly the specialists that you go to (along with optometrists/ophthalmologists and dentists - to treat the eye and mouth symptoms).

I was in the office of the right type of specialist, with four symptoms of the second most common autoimmune disorders and she never thought to ask me if I had dry eyes or dry mouth. I have two and a half pages of her description of my exam from that day and no place in there is there any mention of asking about these things.

Makes me cranky.

Back to 2011. As I mentioned, three days before I found out about the Rheumatoid Arthritis, I got the call that I had a nodule on my thyroid that was 1 inch by 0.5 inch by 0.5 inch. That call came on a Friday and I spent the entire weekend mildly freaked out about it. I read information, I worried, I imagined surgeries and malignancy. It was your pretty typical "diagnosis worry."

Then my doctor called Monday night and told me that I had Rheumatoid Arthritis. All of the sudden the thyroid problem didn't seem so bad. Heck, they can take it out and give me meds to replace what a thyroid does and I can live long and happy. Yes, there are annoying things about it (like when my medication dose isn't quite right and I end up having symptoms of either hypo- or hyperthyroidism), but in general it's definitely minor compared to autoimmune diseases. And even before I had done any research or learned anything else about autoimmune disease, I knew that much was true.

The thyroid surgeries were taken care of first. They took

out the left side that had the nodule. The nodule itself was benign, but they did find malignant cells in the half of the thyroid that came out with the nodule. Four days later I was back in surgery to have the right side out (they always take both sides if malignant cells are found).

A few weeks later, I had my first appointment (really second if you count the one in 2008) with the rheumatologist, Dr. A. I don't remember a whole lot about it (I've had so many rheumatologist appointments by now that they've started to blend together), but I remember being checked for which joints are tender, talking about my fatigue and pain, and being given my first medication.

We never discussed the possibility of another diagnosis. We never discussed what other symptoms I might want to watch for if my condition wasn't neatly described by the diagnosis of RA. We just marched ahead with that diagnosis. When I think about that now, I think it's a little strange - I had been diagnosed simply by the two most generic autoimmune blood markers that could have been there with almost any of the autoimmune diseases and yet it was never questioned that my diagnosis was RA.

I spent March 2011 to January 2013 going from one medication to another when they didn't work, or worse when they caused horrible side-effects or allergic reactions. In all I went through 7 different sets of medications.

I switched to a different rheumatologist in January 2013, when Dr. A stopped practicing in my city (she'd formally worked in two places). In March of 2013 I saw my new rheumatologist, "Dr. B." I went through my history and the list of medications I'd tried in the last two years, none of which had worked. Dr. B suggested that we take a step back - that we redo blood work and take a fresh look at my diagnosis. He felt that I didn't have RA - based on the fact that although I have joint pain, I haven't had joint swelling.

This was the first time that someone had asked me if my eyes and mouth were dry. By this point my eyes were so uncomfortable that I was slowly transitioning from wearing glasses (instead of contacts) only before bed and after I woke up in the morning to wearing them at least half the time. He introduced me to the term "Sjögren's Syndrome" and suggested that I go home and read up on it.

I went down for X-rays of my hands and feet and blood work. Three weeks later I was back in Dr. B's office to discuss the results. I had read information on Sjögren's in the mean-time and I was absolutely convinced that it played a role in what was going on with me, but I still just relegated that disease to dry eyes and mouth. I was certain that something else was going on to cause the fatigue and joint pain. Sjögren's just didn't seem severe enough to be causing all that was going on with me.

Based on the blood work, my history and my symptoms, Dr. B felt that I probably had Sjögren's and may have an overlap of RA or Lupus. This was the first time Lupus had made it's way into discussions of my diagnosis. It was a very scary word as far as I was concerned. In fact I focused on it so much that I think that was part of why I was still in the mindset that the Sjögren's only caused part of my symptoms - I never once considered it could be my only autoimmune diagnosis.

Dr. B sent me to an ophthalmologist for testing to de-termine the extent of my dry eyes and to confirm the Sjögren's diagnosis. And sure enough, the ophthalmologist confirmed it! He tried punctal plugs (basically they plug the hole through which tears drain out of my eye in an attempt to keep the few tears I do produce in my eyes longer). I hated them - I could physically feel them and they caused pressure that gave me headaches. Thankfully they were the kind that dissolved and when I went back in a week to check on them we agreed that they weren't for me. He put me on Restasis eye drops to help with tear production. I was sent out with a prescription and a follow-up appointment in a year.

In the meantime, Dr. B had put me back on the medication that I had taken early on in my first two years after the RA diagnosis. I had been on it for 4 months that time and it hadn't worked for me. He said I needed to be on it longer - like six months - so I went back on it. Along with prednisone.

By that point it was the end of April, 2013.

Musical Diagnosis

I began reporting symptoms in early 2008. I was diagnosed with Rheumatoid Arthritis in March 2011. That's three years of wondering "what is wrong with me?" That's hard on a person. You doubt yourself - are you really feeling these things or is it some kind of personal flaw? Are you really fatigued or are you lazy?

I've read other peoples' descriptions of the relief they felt in finally getting a diagnosis and I agree. Yes, it's a terrible disease and there's a long list of other health problems that I'd trade my autoimmune issues for if I *have* to deal with health issues. But it's still a relief. It affirms that it wasn't all in your head. It gives you something to focus on, to learn about, to conquer. It lets you know what treatment options might be effective. Autoimmune diagnoses do open up a whole new bag of concerns, worries and stresses, but diagnosis is still a welcome event in the process.

So imagine what it's like when you're told that the diagnosis that you've had for two years is likely *not* what's wrong with you at all.

You've focused on that disease - its facts, symptoms, prognosis, and treatments. For two years. You've accepted it and are doing your best to live with it. It's become a part of your identity. You've taken 7 different medicines for that disease - some of which caused you to react badly, and some were wildly expensive.

And now it's gone. It's now added to the original 3 years before the mis-diagnosis. Only worse, actually, because you've invested money, time and your body (by undergoing treatments) in that disease for nothing.

When Dr. B suggested, at my first appointment with him, that I likely did not have RA, I actually felt very defensive. It was a part of me by then, and he was saying it wasn't valid. I started justifying why I felt that I did have it - the pain, the two years of treatment. Surely I wouldn't have been treated for something for two years if it could be discounted as easily as saying "but in all that time you've never had joint swelling - just the pain." If it was that obvious then shouldn't it have been noticed before now? How had I gone this long without that being brought up? That couldn't be right. And therefore I took it defensively, almost personally.

By the second appointment with Dr. B (three weeks after the first), when he began discussing the results of my new blood work, I was ready to accept that maybe there were other issues going on with me. I was pretty sure from the research I'd done in those three weeks that I had Sjögren's Syndrome. But surely that wasn't all of it. Surely there was something more to this joint pain. Maybe I just hadn't developed the hallmark swelling of RA yet. Maybe they'd caught it early enough in my disease progression that it just hadn't happened yet. And besides, everywhere you look information is constantly saying that the reason autoimmune diseases are so complicated is because they can manifest so differently in each person - it's such an individual process.

I was actually more comfortable when he said that he felt I had Sjögren's with a possible RA or even Lupus overlap than when he'd pretty much just said I didn't have RA during the previous appointment.

But then I reacted to this information in a way that was just as strange to me, intellectually, as the defensive way I'd reacted during that first appointment. I didn't want to really tell people that's what was going on with me. When I first got the diagnosis in 2011, I shared it with family and friends. Many had relatives or other friends that had suffered with RA and expressed their sympathy to me. From time to time, I'd share my pain or bad reactions to medication on Facebook or with a friend when they asked, although I had done so more frequently in the beginning than by the time I switched to Dr. B in 2013.

So I felt like people had spent two years aware that I had RA and that I was undergoing various treatments for it. I somehow felt ashamed by now having to say that it had been the wrong diagnosis all along. It somehow felt like the equivalent of raising money by telling people it was for my kid's ball team but then using the money to go shopping for myself. OK, maybe not *that* bad, but that's the general feeling I'd felt – like I'd mislead people.

I felt like I'd cashed in emotional credits for something that hadn't even been wrong with me. I know, intellectually, that life doesn't work that way - that no one would blame me for being misdiagnosed. It's not like it was my fault it happened and I knowingly mislead people. It's not even like I mislead people - I told them the truth as far as I knew it at the time. I expressed my reality to them.

But just because I know things intellectually, that doesn't mean they are the things that influence my thoughts and actions. So whenever someone would ask for an update on what was going on I would casually mention that now I also had this "Sjögren's thing" but "with an overlap of RA and possibly Lupus." And the first part of that sentence was almost always said with a quick, almost "waving it off" attitude, while the last part of the sentence was emphasized. I've slowly got better at this - and being able to publicly write about it is evidence that I have made progress - but I still have this irrational feeling of guilt at "changing my diagnosis."

I'm a mess.

And this game of Musical Diagnoses had another effect on me. I've become wary of diagnoses. Maybe I should have been a little more wary the first time. Maybe I should have asked more questions, sought another opinion, or in some way pressed more to be sure that RA was truly what I had before we proceeded with two years of treatments.

But that's the problem with autoimmune diseases. There's no clear-cut diagnosis method. There's over 80 autoimmune diseases and they mimic each other. They have symptom and blood marker overlap - several different diseases could result in similar blood test results. There are some tests that are more specific for one type of disease - such as the SS-A and SS-B antibody tests for Sjögren's - but even they aren't cut and dry.

Let's use that as an example. (Warning - here comes my math-nerdiness in all its glory!)

SS-A:

- They say 70% of the people that have Sjögren's test positive for this antibody.
- If 4 million Americans have Sjögren's, that means that 2.8 million people will test positive for SS-A.
- But the flip side of that is that 1.2 million people that *have* Sjögren's will *not* test positive for SS-A.

SS-B:

- They estimate 40% of the people that have Sjögren's test positive for this antibody.
- Using the 4 millions American's, that means that 2.4 million Americans that *have* Sjögren's will *not* test positive for this antibody.

So over 2 million people may have a disease even though they have negative results on a blood test for it. I don't know about you, but that's a big chunk of people. I definitely wouldn't want to rule out Sjögren's simply because my blood test was negative - I could be one of those 2 million. (Hence the reason that *all* doctors should ask the simple questions about dry eyes and dry mouth when patients complain of fatigue and joint pain! Those other symptoms may lead to further testing and diagnosis despite a negative anti-body blood test).

So you might be thinking "But you tested positive for both SS-A and SS-B, so you're not one of those people that might be undiagnosed because they have the disease but don't test positive for the antibodies! What are you worried about?"

Well that's true. For Sjögren's. But what about the other antibodies for which I'm currently testing negative that are used to diagnose other autoimmune diseases? Maybe I'm one of the people for *those* diseases that actually has the disease yet doesn't show the blood markers. Or maybe my antibodies just haven't built up enough yet. For example, in 2011 I was negative for anti-dsDNA (another antibody) but in 2013 I was positive for it. Does that mean I had it in 2011 and it just wasn't showing up? Or does that mean that I didn't have it in 2011 but that I do now? Do I even have it now?

At first I was too trusting of my diagnosis. They said I had RA, so OK...that's what I've got and that's what we'll deal with. But, after two years invested in RA, I'm now told that's probably not what I have, it's probably this other thing with maybe this third thing overlapping. I'm starting to move towards the distrusting side - when will I be able to take a diagnosis and feel confident with it? Will I reach a point where I can say "this is what I have" again or will I constantly be worried about new symptoms and new diseases (which could lead you down the slippery slope towards everyone thinking you're a hypochondriac)?

Why does it even matter what my diagnosis is? Many of these diseases are treated with the same drugs (basically that's an artifact of the trial and error with which these diseases seem to be treated). Why does it matter that I know exactly what diseases I have, and if I develop new ones along the way that those are identified as well? Because although they can mimic each other in symptoms, they do have different consequences. For example - RA and Lupus both have joint pain. But RA's joint pain is caused by a process that, if left un-checked, will result in the destruction and distortion of joints (typically seen in the twisted fingers of many sufferers). Lupus does not lead to this. However, Lupus has other consequences for internal organs that need to be monitored (such as kidneys) that are different from RA.

Where's the fine line between being satisfied with a diagnosis enough to feel that settled and relieved feeling that I described earlier that comes with finally having a name for what's going on, and being too settled that you won't notice or find other things that are going on that need attention as well?

Even in the two months since originally writing this chapter and coming back to edit it, more physical symptoms have been noticed by the physicians, more blood tests have been ordered and we're waiting to see if any "overlap diagnoses" are added to my file. Each time a new symptom is found or a new blood test is ordered there's hope that maybe this will be the final piece of the puzzle that leads to definitive diagnosis and a solid treatment plan. However, more often than not it just adds to the layers of unknown.

Second Opinions

As I've stated already, I'm a mess. I have mental blocks that cause me to do or not do things that I know, intellectually, are silly. Yet it doesn't stop them from affecting my behaviors.

One of these mental blocks is seeking a second opinion.

Here's an example of a time that a "second opinion" snuck up me without even really realizing it…and how the "fall-out" was exactly what has kept me from actively seeking second opinions.

In April 2013, after switching to my second rheumatologist ("Dr. B"), I was referred to an ophthalmologist (we'll call him "Dr. O"). Dr. B referred me for dry eye testing to confirm the Sjögren's diagnosis that he suspected from my new blood work. He indicated that Dr. O was someone that has handled many Sjögren's cases and is familiar with the dry eye testing - he said it wasn't difficult but that Dr. O was already familiar with it.

Dr. B did ask if I saw an eye doctor and I said that I did (annual exams for glasses/contacts). He told me that I could go to my regular optometrist but he wasn't sure if my specific one was familiar with the techniques that he was requesting (there's more than one way to test for dry eyes, apparently). I didn't even really think much about it and said that I'd just go to the Dr. O that Dr. B was suggesting, just to make it easier (they've already worked together and we know for sure Dr. O already is familiar with what Dr. B wants him to do).

This exchange never even occurred to me as setting up a "second opinion" circumstance - if it had occurred to me to look at it that way, I probably would have chosen differently because of my "mental block" towards second opinions.

I went to Dr. O, he performed the dry eye testing, confirmed that I did indeed have chronically dry eyes. He placed temporary punctual plugs. A week later I went back and said I hadn't liked the plugs so he gave me a prescription for Restasis and did my field of vision test (one of the medications I'm on for Sjögren's has a side-effect that can damage the eyes - so anyone that is on this specific medication needs annual testing to monitor the eyes for changes). He had me re-book for a follow up appointment in a year.

This all seemed pretty straight-forward and normal to me (well as normal as chronic dry eyes and punctal plugs can be). I never thought anything more about it in terms of which doctor I'd gone to see after that initial conversation with Dr. B.

Then my kids and I went for our annual eye exam at our regular optometrist 4 months later. My kids each had their turn having their eyes checked and updating their prescriptions. Then it was my turn. I sat in the chair and started telling the optometrist about how things had changed since the last time I'd been there. For the previous 24 years, I'd worn contacts and just had a pair of glasses as "back-up" that I only updated every few years.

I let him know that I had been diagnosed with Sjögren's and that I'd gone to an ophthalmologist that I was referred to by my rheumatologist. I told him about the punctal plugs and the Restasis and the order from Dr. O that I not wear contacts because they were beginning to damage my eyes. Mostly I went through all of this because I wanted to let the optometrist know that I wouldn't be needing a contact lens prescription or the "contact lens fitting" that you always have to do.

The optometrist immediately became defensive and indicated that he could have done all of that for me. He had done a special imaging of my eyes in 2011 when I had first gone on the medicine that has possible side-effects related to the eyes (2013 was my second time being on it after it didn't work the first time). In fact he still had those images in my file in front of him. He picked them up and let them drop back to the table and said "Now there's two doctors in the mix with it." He also made some comment about MD's always referring to other MD's because the OD's weren't seen as being as well qualified.

I began to feel pretty anxious at this turn of events. As I mentioned earlier I hadn't even considered that my going to see Dr. O had been a "second opinion." I see lots of specialists. I go to an endocrinologist for my thyroid hormone regulation, a rheumatologist for my autoimmune disease and I've seen various other specialists throughout my life for other issues. When Dr. B referred to me a specialist to have a test done to confirm his diagnosis, I never even considered that it would be viewed in this way by my regular optometrist.

I immediately began to backtrack and muttered my way through some explanation of "I just did what my rheumatologist said to do." It was clear that the optometrist felt his toes had been stepped on and I wanted no part in the blame for that. He was, after all, just about to do an eye exam on me and I prefer to have my medical professionals thinking of me in a positive light while working with me.

This is a beautiful example of why I have the mental block towards second opinions. This had never happened to me before this incident, but yet I always felt like there would be some kind of backlash from seeking a second opinion.

I don't want any "first" doctor to think that I didn't believe/trust/respect/listen to him by my requesting a "second" opinion. Even though it had never happened to me before (mostly because I'd never sought a second opinion for anything in my life), I had always imagined that it would. I imaged that if I then went back to the "first" doctor after having met with the "second" that the "first" would somehow treat me differently. Like he didn't really want to be working with me or like he was thinking "well then why don't you just go to the other doctor if you don't think I'm doing the best for you." I even go so far as to imagine that if I never went back to the "first" doctor - if I continued with the "second" - the "first" doctor would be out there somewhere holding a grudge against me for not coming back.

I'm a non-confrontational person. I'm a pleaser. I don't want anyone to not like me. I don't want anyone to have a reason to not like me. I don't want to make anyone feel badly about themselves. This isn't just about medical professionals - these traits extend to every part of my life.

I hadn't even *meant* to be seeking a second opinion with this ophthalmologist/optometrist thing and I *still* felt the back-lash that I'd feared! And the worse thing about this experience, in August 2013, is that it happened right about the time that I was starting to work up the nerve to seek another opinion on my autoimmune disorders in general.

I had wanted to switch doctors during the second half of 2012. For a variety of reasons, I didn't feel like Dr. A was a good fit for me. I didn't feel listened to and I felt like each appointment was just going through the motions - she would check each joint, and mark down which were tender on her little picture of a skeleton. Then if the medication I was on wasn't working after the necessary amount of time for that specific medication she'd switch me to the next one. But my "second opinion mental block" stopped me from doing anything about it.

Then in January, 2013, Dr. A stopped practicing in my town. That's when I switched to Dr. B - guilt free because I hadn't sought Dr. B while Dr. A had still been a possibility for me.

But in the fall of 2013 I was feeling all the emotions and issues I described in the last chapter, and I was starting to doubt if everything was pinned down just yet. I was also feeling like Dr. B had been very thorough in the beginning (ordered new blood work and x-rays, "stepped back" to look at my diagnosis with fresh eyes, etc.) but that lately things were just on cruise control.

At my appointment with Dr. B in May 2013, we went over the results of my dry eye testing and the notes from my visits with Dr. O. He asked me how I was doing on my medications (I was 2 months into one that needs 6 months to determine if it's effective and I'd been on a low dose of prednisone - something I don't like using - for two months). I indicated that the prednisone had seemed to decrease my pain noticeably. Dr. B told me to go on half dose for a month or two and then go without the prednisone all together and to continue the other one to see if it will work or not. Then he didn't have me re-book. He didn't request a follow-up appointment. It was the first time I'd left a rheumatologists office in 2 years without the doctor saying "set another appointment up for [some length of time] from now."

I thought: "well, maybe he thinks this is going to work." Maybe the prednisone has knocked down the inflammation and pain enough that it won't come back and the other medication will have a chance to kick-in and I'll be stable for a while.

Then I weaned myself off the prednisone and the pain came back - with a vengeance.

I called Dr. B's office, left a message with the nurse and received a call back to go back on the half-dose of prednisone and booked an appointment for over a month later (I had indicated in my message to the nurse that the doctor had not requested that I set up a follow-up appointment so I didn't have one that I could just wait and talk to him about this issue at my next appointment).

This was around the time I started thinking that maybe it was time I make the drive to KU Med - the teaching hospital an hour away.

Then the optometrist appointment happened and I thought "maybe that mental block was right and I should just leave well enough alone and not seek another opinion."

I went to that next rheumatologist appointment in September 2013. By this point I'd been on the autoimmune medication for 6 months. Plus I'd been on it for 4 months in 2011 under Dr. A's care. So here I was, just past the 6 month mark and it wasn't working. If I went off the prednisone, I hurt like crazy. Even with the half-dose that he'd put me back on, it hurt enough to be constantly noticeable and an intrusion in my daily life. In fact, even the full dose that I'd been on for 2 months back in the spring hadn't taken it away - it has just "noticeably reduced" it.

Dr. B's response to me summarizing how I felt on these medications was to say "If you don't think it's working then just stop taking it. You'll know in 6 weeks or so if it had been working or not. Come back in 3 months." (To be fair he said other things, too…those two sentences weren't all he said during the appointment, but that was his recommendations for the immediate future).

By the time I got home, these recommendations/plans weren't sitting well with me. I'll talk about "symptom creep" later, but basically it's very hard to judge exactly how symptoms change over long periods of time. I can tell if I hurt worse today than I did yesterday. But it's hard to accurately judge if on average I hurt worse today than I did on average 6 weeks or 6 months ago. A lot has happened in my life during that time and our memory of things fades and warps.

This "well, just quit taking it and see if you start to hurt worse" wasn't exactly my idea of proactive treatment.

Even at that point, it took me another 4 weeks and two times of talking about it with my therapist before I finally made the call to get an appointment at KU Med. That's how strong my mental and emotional block is towards seeking second opinions.

I know that it's my body, it's my illness, it's my life. I know that I have the right to seek as many opinions as I want. Intellectually, I know that I should not feel bad in the slightest for seeking a second opinion. It's not like I'm "cheating" on anybody. And even if a doctor does take it offensively (like the optometrist did), that shouldn't stop me. I cannot control how other people react to things I do. I can only choose to do things based on my best interest (as long as it's not harmful to others…I understand that you can't take this attitude too far and become completely egocentric!). If a doctor gets offended because I asked someone else for an opinion then that's too bad for them. Actually, they should want me to get the best treatment possible and if they're not the right person for that then they should probably help me find the person or place that is.

In the end, I'm glad I found the "courage" to leave Dr. B and seek out another. I wasn't sure that the "Dr. C" would be "the one" - but at least I'd taken control of my medical care and not continued to be treated by someone that I knew wasn't meeting my needs. I recently read a wonderful book called *The Empowered Patient* by Elizabeth Cohen[*] and it reinforced this feeling. (If anyone is struggling with similar issues as I do with seeking a second opinion, I highly recommend this book!) However, "Divorcing Dr. Wrong" as she puts it still comes with frustrations - I've had to start all over. I spent 8 months with Dr. C and all we did was chase symptoms. We went through test after test, trying to nail down exact diagnoses for all the various symptoms before changing treatment. Some of the tests hadn't been done before, but the first 3 months or so after switching to Dr. C was basically all repeating the same lab work I'd had done with Dr. B and was all in my medical record.

---

[*] http://www.elizabethcohen.com/

We're taught to shop around for so many things – cars, electronics, cell phone providers. *Consumer Reports* magazine is all about giving information to make an informed decision with purchases. However, we assume that we don't need to (or shouldn't) do that with our doctors. We assume that each doctor is as good as the next – that if this one gave me this diagnosis, prognosis, treatment then the next one will, too. After all, don't we want to assume that all doctors are doing the very best to help all patients? Don't we want to assume that they all have the same training and can help us all equally? The truth is that's not the case. There are jerks in medicine just like there are in any customer service department. And there are fabulous, caring, empathetic, "work until we find a solution" people in every field as well. Just because someone is a doctor doesn't make them caring and empathetic. They're human and their personalities and motivations vary just like they do in every other aspect of humanity. We pay them – we employee them for services just as we do an auto mechanic. Only it's infinitely more important – we're working on our body, not our car. So why do we not think we have the right to shop around for a trustworthy doctor with whom we can form a beneficial relationship just as we can for any other service provider?

The Third Opinion

The way Sjögren's was presented to me, and the first thing you read about it when you search online, is that the white blood cells attacking your moisture producing glands leads to dry eyes and dry mouth. In fact, there's a lot of information about how it's often a "secondary" disease - it occurs often in people with other autoimmune diseases...like a bonus add-on but not the main concern. I was convinced I had it the minute I heard about it (based on years of those symptoms), and the blood work and ocular testing confirmed it. But it seemed like an add-on.

My second rheumatologist ("Dr. B") never once presented the idea to me that it may be my *only* diagnosis - that it could be responsible for all the symptoms and complications I was having. Honestly, RA and Lupus sounded much more severe and I had a greater awareness of them and their seriousness, so they were what I focused on. Dr. B treated Sjögren's as an add-on, so I did as well.

I went for my initial visit with a third rheumatologist at University of Kansas Medical Center (KU Med) in October 2013 ("Dr. C"), and that was the first time that someone proposed to me that it very well could be my only diagnosis. He explained that it can go much deeper than just dry eyes and dry mouth. After that first appointment with him, I researched it further. Up to that point, the superficial research I'd done provided information on what it is and that basically the only thing you can do for it is treat the symptoms - treat the dry eyes and dry mouth. It seemed pretty straight-forward and far less concerning than what was going on with the rest of my body, so I looked at the info quickly and moved on.

But once I began thinking of it as possibly my *only* diagnosis, I began to read further about Sjögren's. Like many autoimmune diseases, it can be systemic. That means that it not only affects the moisture-producing glands but also a wide variety of systems in the body.

I went for my follow-up appointment at KU Med with Dr. C in November 2013. The extensive blood work and X-rays showed him (and me) that I don't have RA. I don't have Lupus. I have Sjögren's - and at least for now - that's it.

As I was leaving the appointment, I texted my husband to let him know I was done and headed home. He asked what the news was and I told him Sjögren's was my only diagnosis. He replied "if you don't have RA then what's wrong with your hands?" This is exactly the response I had, along with just about everyone else that I've tried to explain Sjögren's to over the last few months.

I told him Sjögren's was a systemic disease and that it can cause all these other complications. Later that night when we were talking, he said he looked it up online while I was on my way home and at first it just said the info about dry eyes and mouth. Then he noticed that there was a link to more pages of information after that first initial page and when he clicked on that then he began to see where it described the systemic issues of Sjögren's.

The American College of Rheumatology (the association that the doctors working in this area belong to) adds this to the bottom of its description of what Sjögren's is:

> "Complications in other parts of the body can occur. Pain and stiffness in the joints with mild swelling may occur in some patients, even in those without rheumatoid arthritis or lupus. Rashes on the arms and legs related to inflammation in small blood vessels (vasculitis) and inflammation in the lungs, liver, and kidney may occur rarely and be difficult to diagnose. Numbness, tingling, and weakness also have been described in some patients."[*]

They go on to say this later on the page:

> "A vast majority of patients with Sjögren's syndrome remain very healthy, without any serious complications. Patients should know that they face an increased risk for infections in and around the eyes and an increased risk for dental problems due to the long-term decrease in tears and saliva.
> Rarely, patients may have complications related to inflammation in other body systems, including:
> - Joint and muscle pain with fatigue
> - Lung problems that may mimic pneumonia
> - Abnormal liver and kidney function tests
> - Skin rashes related to inflammation of small blood vessels
> - Neurologic problems causing weakness and numbness"

---

[*] http://www.rheumatology.org/Practice/Clinical/Patients/Diseases_And_Conditions/Sj%C3%B6gren_s_Syndrome/

So I guess I'm not in the "vast majority" - I'm in the "rare patient" category. Many other informational sites on Sjögren's talk about the symptoms everyone with it has (dry eyes, mouth, etc.) versus the "serious" or "rare" symptoms. Wohoo…I'm rare! Ummm…I'd rather be normal right about now!

I was much more prepared to accept this singular diagnosis than I was for the previous 6 months - because I finally had a doctor present it to me as a possible only diagnosis, rather than an add-on that causes the obnoxious but not life-changing symptoms of dry eyes and dry mouth.

OK, so great…that's my diagnosis. I'm on board now. How do we treat it (other than eye drops and the medication I'm on to increase saliva production)? An anti-malarial drug called hydroxychlouroquine (brand name is "Plaquenil") is used to treat the systemic aspects of Sjögren's.

I was on Plaquenil for 4 months in 2011 and had been on it for 8 months by the time I saw Dr. C. Nothing. Nada. No relief of my systemic symptoms. In fact I believe they're getting worse over time. What's next? After the second appointment, Dr. C was going to research the findings of the efficacy of treating more severe Sjögren's with other drugs that are being studied for it's use (they're currently used for other autoimmune diseases but haven't become a main treatment option for Sjögren's yet). I prefer this approach over Dr. B's approach of saying "If you don't think it's working for you then stop taking it and come back in 3 months. You'll know if had been working for you in 6 weeks or so of being off of it."

So where I stood in October 2013 was: one diagnosis of Sjögren's that is manifesting itself systemically (and apparently severely compared with most), and on meds that weren't working without any really clear-cut choices to try next.

An invisible disease that no one has heard of, that on the surface appears annoying but not debilitating (yet very much is) and has only one common treatment that apparently doesn't work for me.

And a feeling like life will never feel normal again.

My Scariest Symptom Yet

I'm pretty sure everyone has a strange hair some place on them that grows longer than it should - at least I'd like to think everyone does because I don't want to be the only weirdo out there! Mine is on my right wrist. It's right in the middle of that round bone that sticks out on the outside of your wrist and every so often I'll notice that it's grown long again and pluck it out. What does this have to do with my autoimmune diseases? Nothing, really.

Except that I can't pluck it out any more. And realizing that fact was the first time I noticed the neurological implications of my disease...even though I didn't know that was what I should call it at the time. I can't pinch the goofy hair with enough strength to pull it out. It slides out from between my first finger and thumb. No matter how many times I try.

It may seem like the most trivial thing in all the world, but it has become the symbol of the part of my disease that is the absolute scariest to me. "Makes me break down and cry because I'm so scared" type of scary. "Keeps me up at night worried about it" type of scary.

How in the world could the ability to not pluck out a random hair on my wrist have such an effect on me? Because

I'm losing my fine motor skills and that was the first time I noticed. I'm losing my strength (and I was not the world's strongest person to begin with…in fact, I'm kind of a wimp!). I'm losing my pincer grasp (which I only know the name of because I've had two children and that's one of the things you learn when you have kids and watch them develop!). I have to actively *think* about making my hands do things that should be automatic. Opening things. Washing my hair. Holding the steering wheel. Writing. Typing. Using my phone or iPad (aiming and hitting the spot I meant to hit) has become a challenge. My hands are clumsy - not being able to hold things and move like they should.

Basically my hands don't do what my brain tells them to do.

At first it would happen after I'd "squeezed" something. The very first time it happened was when I was spray painting picture frames for centerpieces for our wedding. That was the summer of 2011 - not long after I'd been diagnosed. Squeezing the spray paint can button led to not being able to move my hands correctly. Then there were the times that I was cooking and squeezed a lemon or something. Afterwards my hands "didn't work right." Same thing when I was stirring something while cooking. Squeezing the spray can on the bathroom cleaner also did it - and when I went to write something on the shopping list a few minutes later I found that I couldn't write correctly. I couldn't hold the pencil correctly. It was like my brain and my hand were completely disconnected.

I stopped taking the low dose (2.5mg) of prednisone after I went to KU Med the first time (October 2013). Part of stopping it was to get a realistic idea of what's going on with me without it - to see if the other medication I've been on for

8 months at that point is doing anything or not. One of the things that I've noticed most prominently since stopping the prednisone is just how prevalent this neurological issue is. It's almost non-stop now. It's no longer happening just after I've squeezed or stirred or gripped something. It's now happening constantly.

This scares the crap out of me. How will I be able to do anything if my hands won't do what my brain tells them? How will I be able to live a normal life? What if this becomes permanent? What if it goes on so long that there's nothing they can do about it?

And what's most scary is that none of the doctors seem to pay any attention to it at all. I told my first rheumatologist, Dr. A, about it when I first noticed it. She didn't even acknowledge it - not a "that's common" or a "that's not really being caused by this, it could be something else going on with you"... nothing. Not even an acknowledgment, really, that she'd even *heard* that I'd said it.

I described it to my second rheumatologist, Dr. B, when I first switched over to him. *Exact same reaction* - or non-re-action, actually. Nothing. No acknowledgment that I'd even described it, let alone that it was something I was concerned about. At that point I was starting to wonder if I was imagining it.

I also described it to the KU med rheumatologist, Dr. C. He did ask me a few questions about the going numb aspect, but said absolutely nothing about the feeling that my hands "don't work right" - that they aren't doing what my brain is telling them to do.

After stopping the prednisone and it becoming a non-stop phenomenon that seems to be getting worse by the day, I began to do more research on it. Apparently there is absolutely a neurological component of Sjögren's syndrome (along with other autoimmune diseases).

> "Neuropathy, which means inflammation and/or damage to the peripheral nerved, can affect patients with Sjögren's. Neuropathy can cause various symptoms, from 'numbness,' to 'coldness;' in its most severe form, neuropathy has been described as 'burning,' 'lancinating' or 'feeling like my skin is on fire.' Neuropathy can also cause weakness and clumsiness." [*]

It's amazingly frustrating to me that a description that fits what I'm feeling so well is right there, associated with the disease I'm now diagnosed with and yet three doctors have glossed over it (or even out-right ignored it) when I brought it up. How can three doctors ignore what has become the absolute scariest thing I think I've ever had happen to me in my life?

---

[*]   http://www.hopkinsSjögrens.org/disease-information/ Sjögrens-syndrome/neurologic-complications/

Neuropathy Testing

Writing the previous chapter helped me be determined to address my neurological issues at my next doctor's appointment. During my second appointment with Dr. C (November 2013), I talked for quite a while about my neurological concerns. The dexterity problems, weakness, clumsiness, "hands not doing what my brain tells them to do" issues that concern me the most. He referred me for neurological tests to document these things in a way that insurance will allow us to seek treatments that they'd otherwise fight. Apparently insurance thinks of Sjögren's as only a eye/mouth issue as well.

I went to the neurologist for an EMG (electromyography) and NCS (nerve conduction study). The purpose of these procedures was to test for, and document, neuropathy.

The nurse conducted the NCS first. They stick various sensors on you and zap you in places with electricity to measure how long it takes the electricity to travel down your nerves to a sensor.

It hurts.

In reading about the test beforehand, people likened it to a static electricity shock that you get in the winter. Ummm…

not quite. A lot worse.

One time when I was teaching chemistry, I was demonstrating to my students how to use a conductivity tester. Like a dummy, I washed it off and tilted it in a way that the tester shocked me. And this was not the 9-volt battery-operated kind, it was the plug-into-a-regular-electrical-outlet kind. I jerked back, dropped the tester and broke the light bulb. It hurt like crazy and I thought "man, that was dumb of me!"

That's what this felt like. Over and over, directly on my nerves to measure how fast it would travel.

Made me cry.

Then the doctor came in to do the EMG. He introduced himself, talked about what he was going to do - explained why it's not that bad. He said the needles were very thin - like acupuncture - and that it's much easier than drawing blood because it goes into the muscle and any part of the muscle will do. You don't have to "thread the needle" like you do with drawing blood - he said it's more like hitting the side of a barn with a baseball. He even made a point to explain how he had to do the procedure on himself before he could do it on patients and how he learned what made it hurt and how to make it not hurt.

OK…sounds alright so far.

Until he started. OUCH!

The needle in the muscle is uncomfortable but definitely bearable. But then he would ask me to move in various ways (flex my foot, tighten a specific muscle, etc.) to see how the muscles reacted to the signals to move or contract. That's when it really hurt.

The needle is in the muscle that was being moved…and when I moved the muscle the needle moved, too. Holy heck that hurt! Especially the needle on the top of my foot!

After he was done, he had me sit up and proceeded to tell me that everything was fine. All the results of both tests were normal.

So I asked him why was this was all going on with me?

He began to explain that everyone, when they are immobile in the wrong position, has limbs that go to sleep. He used the example of people holding their cell phones to their ear to talk and their hands going numb. I explained that I have this dexterity problem all the time - mobile or immobile. And I explained how they don't work right - loss of fine motor skills, etc.

He explained *again* that when anyone is immobile in the wrong position they have limbs go to sleep. And he explained *again* that this was good news - that I didn't have any permanent damage to my nerves and therefore my Sjögren's wasn't getting worse.

First: wasn't getting worse? How can he say that when even in just the last 3-4 months I've noticed a sharp decline in my health and ability to function.

Second: which part of "happens even when I'm mobile" did he not understand? I understand that when you sit or hold a limb in the wrong position it falls asleep…everyone understands and experiences that, but this is *different.*

It's constant, continual and doesn't matter if I'm moving or not. It's happening while I'm typing this. It happened when I drove to pick up my kids a few hours ago. It happened when I was eating lunch right after that doctor's appointment. And it happens many, many times each day.

The look on his face when he declared me "perfectly fine" and when I asked him why was this all going on with me was very clear to me. He thought this was all in my head. He explained it away to himself as a silly woman that didn't realize that when you sit in a funny position for too long your limbs go to sleep. He clearly felt that I should be thrilled with his proclamation of "everything's fine!" and jump with joy and go out the door on my merry way.

While I was eating lunch 15 minutes later (obviously not being immobile), I had to actively concentrate to be able to pick up the french fries between my first and second finger and my thumb. I should not have to actively concentrate to perform such a task!

All it would have taken for me to have had a very different experience at that appointment would have been for the doctor to say "I understand that you're having these symptoms and that they're very concerning for you. The tests that we've done today don't show the reason that you're experiencing it. The good news is that the disease hasn't caused any permanent nerve damage, but unfortunately the bad news is that this information isn't explaining why you're experiencing these problems. I suggest that you talk with your rheumatologist more to try to find out why you're experiencing these things."

I have no problem with his interpretation of the test

results showing that, as far as they can determine, he can't find out what's causing this. That's fine with me. I'm not upset that these results didn't show a clear cause.

I am, however, extremely upset with the glib attitude he had. With the attitude that obviously the only explanation for what's going on with me is that I sit immobile in the same spot too long.

And I am upset that when I tried to explain to him that it is more than that, he simply repeated the exact same explanation to me again.

I know there is more than sitting immobile in an awkward position wrong with me. I know that I am losing fine motor capabilities. I know that I continually have to actively concentrate on tasks with my hands that should be completely automatic. I know that I have to stop doing something to shake my hands in an attempt to "shake it out." I know that I have weakness and clumsiness that is not normal. I know that after I was scrubbing the shower (obviously not immobile), when I went to the other room to add a cleaning supply to the shopping list, my hand wouldn't work and I couldn't write the words on the list. I know that many times, when I sign my name on a credit card slip, it's harder to do, takes more concentration, and looks less and less like "my signature."

And I know that it is absolutely possible, and necessary, for doctors to show more compassion and empathy for their patients than that one did that day with me.

At my third appointment with the rheumatologist (Dr. C) after this experience with the neurologist, I was better able to communicate just exactly what's going on with fine motor skills and that prompted concerns of central nervous system involvement, which lead to an MRI to look for lesions in the white matter of my brain and have an appointment with a (different!) neurologist for a full neurological workup. Following that, Dr. C said he'd likely start me on an infusion drug that is taken through IV once, then again two weeks later. He said he hoped it will last 6-12 months at a time.

However, despite months of testing, learning to be much more exact and informative in my description of these symptoms, correcting doctors when they describe the symptoms inaccurately back to me, and appointment after appointment, I'm still chasing this fine motor control/dexterity issue – both trying to get doctors to accurately understand what it is that I feel and trying to figure out what's causing it.

The Medications Carousel

Along the road to diagnosis, I have been riding on a medications carousel.

When I was first diagnosed, everyone said "It's not like it used to be - there's so many more medications available now than ever before…it's much easier to treat than it used to be." That gave me hope and helped keep my attitude positive.

At least that's what happened when I was diagnosed with RA. When I was diagnosed with Sjögren's, everyone just said "What's that?" and "How do they treat that?" Far less hope-inducing.

4 years and 7 sets of drugs later, including two allergic reactions, one that I couldn't tolerate and none of which worked for me, that hope that was given to me with the prospect of better medications is pretty much gone.

In fact, whenever I see one of those commercials on TV with people happily going about their life while on a new auto-immune drugs, it just makes me cranky…been there, done that, didn't work!

As if the medication carousel wasn't bad enough in its

own right, now that my diagnosis has changed, many of these were experiences that I wouldn't have had to go through if I had I been diagnosed correctly years ago.

For those that aren't familiar with the types of medications used for autoimmune diseases, there are three main types - steroids, NSAIDs (non-steroid anti-inflammatory drugs) and DMARDs (disease modifying antirheumatic drugs).

Steroids and NSAIDs attempt to reduce inflammation throughout the body but do nothing to treat the underlying processes of the diseases. DMARDs attempt to modify the disease process itself - and in the processes of doing this, the symptoms will hopefully be relieved as well.

They're often used in conjunction, using the NSAIDs to calm the current symptoms while the DMARDs have a chance to work. I was on several NSAIDs over the course of the years (none have helped), but this description will focus on the DMARDs.

I began my first medication in April 2011 with Dr. A for the diagnosis of RA. Her philosophy on medication was to start with those that have been used the longest.

All of these medications come with side-effects, many of which are significant, and she felt it was better to start with the meds that had been used the longest as she knows the most about what those side-effects are and I could be monitored for them. All of these drugs were accompanied by blood work every month or two (depending on how long I'd been on the particular drug) to monitor for various side-effects (kidney and liver function, etc.)

The descriptions that are below are my personal experiences. Many people have found great relief from one or more of the medications I have been on. I share this information not to discourage anyone's use of any medication that they and their doctor feel would benefit them. I'm sharing this so people can get an understanding of the mental, emotional and physical drain that the medicine carousel causes.

I also describe my struggles with doctors, insurance companies, pharmacies and other aspects of treating a chronic disease.

1. Sulfasalazine (brand name Azulfidine)

My first medication was sulfasalazine. It's a medication that you have to work your way up to therapeutic dosage. For the first week I took one pill each evening. During the second week I took one in the morning and one in the evening. As these two weeks progressed, I felt that I was getting worse. My fatigue and joint pain were worsening and by the end of the second week, the base of my skull was extremely tender. It reminded me of when lymph nodes are swollen when you're sick, but it was in the back of my skull. I had looked for information about it over the weekend and saw that worsening symptoms are sometimes the result of allergic reactions to the medication.

I called Dr. A and left a message with her nurse describing what was going on with me. This was the morning that I was to take 2 pills in the morning and 1 in the evening (eventually the goal was 2 morning and 2 evening). I took the 2 pills that morning like I was supposed to do. Later that morning, the nurse called me back to explain that the medication was not what was making me worse and that RA doesn't affect the neck or head (clearly implying that these symptoms I called and left a message about were not related to my RA nor the medication that I was on). She left a message for me because I wasn't able to get to my phone in time.

By this time I was itching all over - crazy itching. I called her back and let her know about this itching all over and after consulting with the doctor she let me know that I was allergic to the medication and I was to discontinue taking it and she would put a note of the allergy in my file.

2. Hydroxychloroquine (brand name Plaquenil)

The second medication I was put on was hydroxychloroquine. It's an anti-malarial drug that is routinely used for autoimmune diseases. I was told it would take 4-6 months to even tell if it was going to work.

There's an especially cruel nature to the medications used for autoimmune diseases - they all take time to know if they're even going to work. For some medications that time period is 3-4 months, for others it's 4-6 months. So each time you're switched to a new medication you know that there is going to be a period of time (that is months long) that you will have no effect. And that if after the "waiting period" it doesn't work, you'll just have to go through another "waiting period" with the next drug. You wait for 6 months to find out that something doesn't work for you, and then have to start another 4-6 month period to wait and see if the next one works.

This time I didn't have any bad effects, but it just didn't work. I was on it for 4 months and saw nothing from it.

3. Methotrexate (brand name Trexall)

Next came a cancer drug, methotrexate. In fact, I saw a cartoon not long ago that shows a patient in a doctor's office and the doctor says "The good news is that it's not cancer. However the bad news is that it's autoimmune disease and you'll be on chemotherapy for the rest of your life." That cartoon was likely talking about methotrexate.

It's a drug that has much more serious side-effects than the first two I'd been on. Including that you CANNOT drink alcohol while on it. I'm not a big alcohol drinker - maybe a drink or two a month, some months without any. But the reason this made me sad was not only that it's taking away freedoms in my life, but because I was switching to this drug right before I was getting married.

I chose to wait until after the wedding to switch to it so I could enjoy a drink or two at the party with my new husband. But our honeymoon wasn't going to happen until a month later and I'd already been on this carousel for 6 months and I wanted to get going on this new medication. So that meant that I spent the 5 days on a semi-private island off the coast of Belize not being able to enjoy a single drink from the free island tiki bar! Free, frozen, fruity drinks available any time I wanted (and those are my favorite kind!) and I couldn't have any at all. It was definitely a bummer.

This was also a drug that I needed to work up to full dose with, and by the time I was at full dose I realized I was not able to tolerate the drug. I felt like a zombie. I have fatigue from the disease, but this added a whole other level - I couldn't get up, couldn't keep my eyes open, couldn't think about anything. I couldn't function in life at all.

In a report from Dr. C's office to my PCP, there is a description of my history of medications. One sentence says "She failed methotrexate." This may be very common medical speak, but I don't think it should be. I didn't fail the medication. The medication failed to help me because I couldn't tolerate it. But just that phrasing implies that it was my fault. And even if the doctors don't believe it's my fault, why use language that implies it? Why set people up to think in this way?

4. Adalimumab (brand name Humira)

Dr. A thought it was time to try the biologics. The biologics are the newest class of drugs for autoimmune diseases and are either injections or infusions. The first (and only, at least so far) biologic class I was on was the TNF-inhibitors.

It took 2 months from the time the doctor prescribed it to me and many, many, many phone calls to actually get my first dose of the drug. It's expensive, very expensive, and insurance companies don't like to pay for it.

My prescriptions are filled through the pharmacy named "Caremark" and my prescription insurance is through the insurance company named "Caremark." One would think that those two entitles would be able to communicate with each other. However, it took at least a dozen phone calls (all of which involved long wait times) to get the pharmacy side to get the correct authorization from the insurance side to fill the prescription.

Yes, both under the same parent company - the insurance side wasn't communicating effectively with the pharmacy side to provide the needed authorization.

I would call one side and they'd tell me it was a problem with the other. I'd call the second side and they'd tell me it was a problem with paperwork from the doctor's office. Then I'd call the doctor's office and they'd tell me the problem wasn't on their end. This went round and round until I was frustrated beyond belief. I felt like I needed to conference call them all in to talk about it with all the parties at the same time - but I couldn't!

I don't even know what I would have done if I hadn't had a job that enabled me to make these phone calls and sit on hold for long periods of time. My previous job as a high school teacher would not have afforded me that ability and I'm sure the process would have dragged on even longer.

In the meantime, I called Dr. A to complain about pain and was given a pain medication.

I finally received my first dose, was trained on how to self-inject the medication and began my every-other-week injections.

First of all, those injections HURT!!!!! The medication is very viscous and must be kept refrigerated (increasing the viscosity). I would sit at my kitchen counter and pep-talk myself into doing it. I'd hold the injection pen (similar to an Epi-pen) on my leg with my finger on the button and tell myself "do it" at least 10 times before I'd actually press the button.

Three months later, the drug wasn't doing anything for me. Dr. A said to increase the dosage to every week instead of every two weeks.

A month later, still no effect.

5. Etanercept (brand name Embrel)
The next TNF-inhibiting biological self-ejector (weekly injection) I was placed on was etanercept. This was Spring 2012 - a year after being diagnosed.

I'm not sure if it was the medication or the fact that it was summer or a small release in the intensity that happens in the ebb and flow that occurs with these diseases, but for a while I felt better. *Not normal. Not good.* But "I can see a light at the end of the tunnel" better.

This lasted about 4 months and then I began going back downhill again. Joint pain and fatigue were becoming more severe - worse than when the journey began in Spring of 2011.

6. Certolizumab pegol (brand name Cimzia)
In December of 2012, I let Dr. A know that I had definitely gone back to hurting and was in fact worse than when I'd started and wanted to know what was next.

This time it was put on certolizumab pegol, an every-other-week TNF-inhibitor injection that was a traditional syringe (the other two had both been the self-injector "pens"). At first I thought I'd hate that, but I actually liked it. I could control how fast it was going in as opposed to the pens that just shoved it all in at once and you had no way to slow it down or pause to take a breath. That did help with the pain of injection.

The first injection seemed OK. I had injection-site reaction (a red, itchy welt at the site of the injection - lasting a couple of weeks after each one) but I'd had that with the other two indictable medications as well and it's common with these drugs.

Two weeks later I did my second injection and I remember feeling nauseous right after - but just a little, not terribly bad. I remember thinking "there's no way that's due to the meds, I just (30 seconds early) injected it into my leg - it couldn't cause nausea that quickly!

I went to see Dr. A the week after that second shot. She asked how it was going, I said fine, she said "it's too early to tell if it's working yet but your blood work doesn't show anything harmful going on, so to keep taking the medication."

A week later I was ready to give injection #3. I put the kids to bed (my husband was playing in his weekly pool league so he wasn't home) and went into the bathroom to do the injection. I sat and prepared the injection site and syringe. I injected it like always.

Within 20 seconds I had extreme nauseousness, ridiculous vertigo and I couldn't hear anything at all. I stumbled my way from the bathroom to the bed (I think I fell once) and climbed into bed. I was completely panicked. I've never felt this way in my life. And it happened literally within *seconds* of injecting the meds. As I lay in my bed I realized my cell phone was still in the bathroom.

I was terrified that I would have to call out to my then-9-year-old son in the next room for him to call 911 for me. I was almost ready to do just that when I realized that it was beginning to fade, ever so slightly. I decided to wait it out and see if it was going to get a little better. Within 30 minutes I could get up and go back to the bathroom to get my phone and quickly finish my bedtime routine.

The vertigo and nausea lasted for a couple of weeks. It would come and go but was definitely a factor in my life for about two weeks. This is the problem with injectable drugs that last for multiple weeks - not only do the benefits last for a few weeks at a time, but any side effects also last!

Unfortunately, this happened just as I was switching doctors. Dr. A had been practicing in my town one day a week and another town the rest of the time but had recently decided to drop the one day a week in my town. That's when I switched to Dr. B.

I called Dr. B's office first thing in the morning and left a message for the nurse. I explained that I had not yet seen Dr. B but that Dr. A would be sending my records over and requesting that Dr. B's office schedule an appointment for me. I described my reaction from the night before and asked what I should do. I obviously was never going to take that medication again, but I wanted to know if that would mean they needed to schedule an appointment for me sooner than if they'd thought I was happily proceeding on that medication (this was my hope, at least).

Later that afternoon they returned my call and let me know that since I wasn't officially a patient of Dr. B's yet that I needed to contact Dr. A to manage my care. So I called Dr. A's office and left a message with the nurse describing what was going on. I got a call back saying that I shouldn't take that medicine anymore (as if I would!) and to wait for Dr. B's office to get my records, schedule me an appointment and call me back. Great. Just want I wanted to hear after that terrible night of a bad reaction…"wait"!

7. Prednisone and Hydroxychloroquine

After the scary bad reaction, I was on no medication at all from January 2013 to April 2013 when Dr. B changed my diagnosis and put me back on hydroxychloroquine. I'd been on it 4 months in 2011 and he said that wasn't long enough to be able to tell so he put me back on it for a minimum of 6 months.

That was April 2013 and I'm still on it in November 2014, although it's doing nothing noticeable for me.

The Letters

I didn't realize, and I would guess most people don't either, that every time you see a specialist they send a letter back to your primary care physician. I first realized this in 2011 when I asked my PCP's nurse to copy any information from my first visit with a rheumatologist in 2008. I expected to receive copies of the lab results and notes from my PCP about why I was being referred to the specialist.

Instead I received a copy of the letter from Dr. A to my PCP. This is the one that I've mentioned before that gave written proof that I had two symptoms of autoimmune disease in 2008 (although I actually had four at the time).

I never really thought about these letters again until recently. When I began seeking care at KU Med, shortly after my first visit, I received a copy by mail of the letter sent to my PCP. This one was primarily written by the resident physician that conducted most of my appointment. It had a portion written by the attending as well.

Despite the paper that I prepared to give the doctors during this visit that listed all of my relevant lab tests, the dates of each medication I was prescribed and the reactions to those medications, there were still errors in the letter. For example,

I had verbally corrected the resident several times when he would say that I'd been on prednisone back in 2011. I had not. The first time I was placed on prednisone was spring of 2013. Even after at least 2 verbal corrections and the written paper I'd brought, the letter to my PCP still indicates that I was on prednisone in 2011 in the "patient history" section (I wasn't on prednisone until 2013). It also indicated that I "didn't tolerate methotrexate and Humira" when it was only the methotrexate that I didn't tolerate - the Humira I was fine taking, it just didn't do anything beneficial for me.

The resident also indicated that the "assessment and plan" for my Sjögren's Syndrome was "take pilocarpine and Rhinocort aqua." The pilocarpine is to help produce saliva - and it works well. But the Rhinocort aqua is my allergy medicine that I take seasonally. It has nothing to do with my Sjögren's. I think he mean Restasis (the eye drops to help reduce inflammation and therefore encourage more tear production).

In the "Attestation" section written by the attending doctor, he indicates "No tender points on examination" which isn't true - most of my finger and toe joints were tender when he pressed on each one during the examination.

The letter from my second visit at KU Med (only the attending was present at that appointment) contained errors as well. This one included sections for past medical history, past surgical history and family history. The surgical history indicated I had a thyroidectomy only the left - when in fact I had the left removed and then 4 days later the right.

In the "History of Present Illness" section it indicates that I "had punctal plugs of [my] lacrimal glands, which has helped to some extent." Wrong. I had them for a week - they were the dissolving kind - and they caused me physical pressure and discomfort so I never had the permanent ones placed it. I clearly explained this to him, yet it appears in the documentation as I currently have them and they're helping.

It also describes my "having persistent numbness and tingling of her upper and lower extremities as well." It then says I have "no other complaints at the current time." That's also incorrect. Yes, I did discuss the numbness – but not numbness and tingling like your arm is asleep, numbness like you've been outside in the cold and come inside and can't write normally because you're hand is cold. I spent far greater time discussing the loss of fine motor control and clumsiness - which to me is an important part of the description of my problems – than "numbness". And I also told him I didn't have any tingling (he had specifically asked).

If all of these errors are made by the specialists as they communicate their encounters with me to my PCP, are these errors affecting my care and treatment? If these errors occurred in the 3 rheumatologist letters that I've received, how many are in the many, many other letters from Dr. A and Dr. B that I never received? If these errors are a part of my documented medical record, will they affect medical or insurance decisions in the future? And why don't all specialists send a copy of the letters to the patient after each visit?

Writing My Own Letter

In May 2014 I went for my scheduled appointment with the Rheumatologist, Dr. C. The appointment was scheduled in February. At the February appointment, he told me that his plan was to order Rituxan as treatment for my Sjögren's (sicca symptoms, fatigue, etc.) after he got the results back from the muscle biopsy I was about to have. He specifically told me that he'd order the treatment no matter if the biopsy results came back positive or negative. He had me schedule this follow-up appointment for May with the understanding that when the biopsy results came back he'd order the treatment and I'd probably be on this infusion for a little while before this follow-up appointment came around.

He thought I was going to have a skin biopsy to test for small fiber neuropathy (since the EMG/NCS was normal and it can miss small fiber neuropathy) the next week. But the neurologist and I both decided that I didn't have the symptoms of small fiber neuropathy (tingling and numbness) - I have fine motor control and muscle weakness issues.

So I was scheduled with neurology for a muscle biopsy (bicep) instead. The biopsy was scheduled 3-4 weeks out and I was told the results would be back in 4-8 weeks. That meant a possible three month "turn-around" from the time I saw Dr.

C in February and set the "plan" and when the biopsy results would be back. I called the rheumatology nurse and let her know this (since it was different from the skin biopsy timeline he'd discussed with me in February) and asked if he could order the treatment without waiting for the results since he was going to do it no matter what the biopsy results were. She said nope; he wanted to wait.

So I had the biopsy and waited to hear back from neurology with the results.

I went for the "follow-up" appointment with rheumatology in May and the first thing he said when he sat down was "well, since the muscle biopsy came back negative - all normal..." to which I looked shocked and said "well, it's nice to finally hear those results since this is the first I've heard of them!" He asked if neurology hadn't communicated the results, and I told him that they most certainly had not, despite me calling a few weeks earlier to check on them.

He then proceeded to tell me that he didn't feel like I warranted the Rituxan treatment. This was after almost 8 months with many appointments with him. At EACH and EVERY appointment he made sure that I understood that Rituxan was the ultimate "goal" treatment and that he was doing more and more tests to rule out other causes of my symptoms before he began the treatment.

So after almost 8 months of appointments leading up to it, he said "that would be like killing an ant with a sledge hammer." This despite him proposing it for all these months of appointments, beginning with the very first time I saw him when he said he was going to go look into the research on it being used with Sjögren's patients.

I began to discuss with him my fatigue and how pervasive it is - how concerning it is when combined with the thought of having to go back to a job like teaching full time (which is far more physically demanding and which I'm pretty certain I'd have a hard time doing if I could even do it at all) when my current flexible jobs ends in a year - which is far more concerning than he seemed to think it was.

At this point he said he'd talk with my primary care doctor and discuss her putting me on stimulants to help keep me awake. Ummmm...nope, not what I want to do. Just helping me "get through" tired moments without treating the underlying problem is not what I'm looking for if there are other possibilities out there that may treat the actual problem. And he never did make that call anyway, despite his follow up letter from the visit saying he would do so.

He still just told me to stay on the same treatment I'd been on for the past year (Plaquenil) that isn't alleviating my symptoms AT ALL and come back in 4 months. Why would I come back in 4 months? I've been coming for almost 8 months and nothing has been treated or managed in any way. I've been on this same medication for over a year and it's not helping. It's not going to be any different 4 months from now!

He said that "of course you're welcome to get a second opinion" and "most doctors wouldn't have gone as far as I have with the testing." So in other words I should be thankful that I went through months and months of testing to eliminate all the other possible causes of my symptoms to have it confirmed that it is, in fact, my currently diagnosed disease (Sjögren's) that's causing the problem only to be told that he's not going to change my treatment plan (despite saying that he was for the past many months) even though it's not working?

I left his office and sat in my car in the parking garage and cried. Ugly, all-out, sobbing cry. I've waited for so many months to rule out other diagnoses to begin treating this one and then it was all taken away.

Then I had to drive an hour home and pack my kids up for my daughter's last dance competition and my son's first baseball tourney of the season - which we had to leave town for within a few hours of me getting home from that appointment. I didn't have time to deal with it. I didn't have time to process it. I had to hold it all together to get through that weekend of both their activities...and then the following week of end-of-school activities and then the following two weeks of a demanding work schedule (running a once-a-year two-week institute for the participants in the science education grant-funded program I managed). And the day that my "two weeks" of crazy ended my son had another baseball tournament beginning. And add to all of this that I had three ophthalmologist appointments during this time - collagen punctal plugs (dissolve after a few days - "trial run"), regular punctal plugs (had in for 9 days and still couldn't stand them - felt them against my eyeballs all the time) and internal punctal plugs - wiped out of my eyes within an hour of having them put in.

All told, it would three and a half weeks from the time I left that appointment until I can breath, take time and really process all of it. I simply couldn't stop right then. I had to be their mom. I had to do my job. I had to get to June 9th. Then I would get a break and deal with the emotions that I was barely keeping under control right then.

And after I processed the emotions, I needed to analyze

my choices for moving forward - which included staying with this doctor and this treatment, seeking another opinion from someone at the same facility or seeking another opinion from someone in another location (which would include significant travel as I feel like I've exhausted resources where I live).
I was barely hanging on - managing to get through the minimum I needed to get through during those few weeks of "holding it together until I got a break". And then one night, about halfway through, I walked into the kitchen after a 10.5 hour day of traveling and work before I went to an 8pm baseball game for my son - and I opened a letter from KU Med that was sitting on the kitchen counter.

It was a copy of the letter from Dr. C to my PCP describing our last appointment. The letter indicated that he felt my fatigue was due to depression, supported by the fact that I was "very tearful and exited the room" during the appointment. Note that he has never done any sort of screen or assessment, nor asked me about, depression.

I was livid. I was appalled. I was hurt. I was crushed. I was outraged. And I had to fight back the tears, get in the car and go to the baseball diamonds. The ballgame did help take my mind off of it for an hour and a half (I LOVE watching my son and his teammates play ball!) but as soon as the game was over it all came crashing back over me like a wave.

And after sleeping on it overnight, below is my response - a letter I wrote (and sent) to my rheumatologist, Dr. C:

Dear "Dr. C,"

I have never in my life questioned what a doctor said. I've never written to a doctor. I've always been a "good patient" and never in any way confronted something that I felt wasn't right. I say that only to let you know how strongly I must be feeling to write this letter. The first portion discusses my reaction to my latest appointment while the second portion discusses the information I've gathered relevant to treating Sjögren's with Rituxan.

I received my copy of the visit letter from my last appointment sent to my new primary care doctor today. I was absolutely appalled to see that you insinuated that I was depressed and that was the cause of my chronic fatigue. Sjögren's, the disease for which you confirmed my diagnosis, is well documented in the medical literature as having chronic fatigue as one of its most debilitating symptoms. (I have read many such articles – such as Segal et al. in 2008 Arthritis Rheumatology entitled "Prevalence, Severity and Predictors of Fatigue in Sjögren's Syndrome" – they found "Abnormal fatigue defined as a FSS score of greater than or equal to 4 was present in 67% of the patients." Or Ng and Bowman in the 2010 Rheumatology article: "Chronic fatigue is one of the most prevalent and debilitating symptoms in primary SS (pSS). Approximately 70% of pSS patients suffer from disabling fatigue, which is associated with reduced health-related quality of life.")

The reason that I was "very tearful" and "left the room" has zero to do with depression. I see a therapist regularly as I deal with the issues that having a chronic, invisible illness causes in a young person's life and she would be more than willing to confirm that my fatigue is not caused by depression. I actually have a very high level of motivation and desire to continue my work and activities but am physically unable to do so. That is not characteristic of depression-caused fatigue but is actually in line with the fatigue as documented in the Sjögren's medical literature. (For example, Gadaert et al. showed in a 2002 Annals of the New York Academy of Sciences that "[Sjögren's patients and healthy participants] did not differ with respect to average levels of reduced motivation or mental fatigue. Both general and physical fatigue and reduced activity varied significantly during the day." Or the Segal paper that found "While fatigue is associated with depression, depression is not the primary cause of fatigue in Primary Sjögren's Syndrome.")

The reason that I was upset was because of the 180-degree change that you'd made in my treatment plan. From the first visit with you, seven months ago, you discussed Rituxan. I had not previously looked into the treatment. You indicated that you would look at the literature and we would discuss it at my second appointment. From that second appointment forward, each and every appointment including you indicating that Rituxan treatment was where we were headed but that you wanted to do various testing, send me to other places, etc., to rule out other causes of my symptoms.

In fact, at my last appointment, in February of 2014, you specifically told me that you would order the Rituxan treatment no matter what the results of the biopsy, but that you wanted to wait until the biopsy results were back before doing so. You even explained to me the process - that once you ordered it, the insurance would need to approve it and then the infusion treatment center would be pretty quick about getting me in - I believe you said I would be in about a week after the approval went through. That appointment left no doubt in my mind that you had every intention of ordering Rituxan - as you specifically said - no matter the result of my biopsy.

To come back 3 months later (and get biopsy results from you that I'm hearing for the first time because apparently neurology doesn't feel it necessary to share those results with me when they got them), and be told that you felt it completely inappropriate to order Rituxan in my case was an enormous shock. If you felt it was so unwarranted then why had you discussed it at each and every appointment with me for 7 months? Why had at the previous appointment you specifically said you would be ordering it no matter the results of my biopsy?

If you changed your mind for some reason, then fine, but explain that. Explain to me why after 7 months of heading towards that treatment you feel it's no longer warranted when my symptoms are the same as they were when I first came to you. Instead, you acted as if I was completely off base expecting that treatment to be ordered - you acted as if you'd never once discussed it with me as something that was actually going to happen. It was if all my previous appointments and conversations with you were completely forgotten.

You also treated my chronic fatigue, which is absolutely the most debilitating symptom of this disease, as if it was inconsequential and like it was something to be envied - you "wished you got as much sleep as me" you said - instead of something that is a major roadblock in my life, family and career.

To realize that after 3 years of no diagnosis at all, and then 2 years of a mis-diagnosis (RA) which lead me through 7 drug treatment plans that were ineffective because they were treating a disease I didn't have, to go through 7 months of appointments with you that I believed were leading to this treatment being ordered (because you explicitly said so) - only to walk in and have you act like you had no idea why I would be expecting it was absolutely shocking to me.

That was why I was tearful and left - because you minimized my fatigue and acted like 7 months of appointments where you'd suggested and discussed the treatment never happened.

As for the feeling that my symptoms do not warrant Rituxan, I do disagree with that. In addition to the citations above (I'm a scientist and PhD that is employed at a research university that gives me access to full articles in peer-reviewed journals – I review the research myself before making decisions), the following lead me to believe that it is worth trying:
One of the first things you see when you Google "Rituxan" and "Sjögren's" is a recent study that is purported to show that Rituxan is ineffective in treating Sjögren's. This article is the latest and "seems" to disagree with previous research showing that Rituxan is indeed effective for Sjögren's.

However, that article is merely a summary of the original research article. When reading the full original research article (Devauchelle-Pensec et al. in the 2014 Annals of Internal Medicine), I found the following:

- Randomized, double-blind, placebo-controlled trial
- There was a significant difference in VAS fatigue score at week 6 (p < 0.001), week 16 (p = 0.012) and even at week 24 (where p = 0.105) there was an almost 50% improvement in the VAS fatigue score.
- Dryness improved by week 24 with p = 0.08
- Their definition of "successful" was >30mm change in >2 of the 4 VAS scores.
- They report that improvement in fatigue and dryness was significant – just not at the 30mm mark that they'd set.
- One of their self-reported weaknesses in their study is that "This primary outcome may have been insensitive to detect clinically important changes in symptoms." (p. 238)
- "Fatigue, which is a major source of disability in patients with primary Sjögren's Syndrome, was the symptom that responded best to rituximab therapy in our study." (p. 238)

Clearly they found clinically significant differences in reduction of both fatigue and dryness. Even a p of 0.105 for fatigue improvement at week 24 is well worth it to someone struggling with daily, life-altering fatigue. The p value, when representing an almost 50% improvement in the symptoms is significant in real life, even if it doesn't meet the p<0.05 significance standards (which is an arbitrary line that has been drawn in the sand anyway). As someone struggling with a disease (that also happens to understand significance testing), I'd take a p of 0.08 or 0.105 any day over doing nothing to attempt to alleviate such pervasive symptoms!

Why I Don't Like to Cover up Pain and Symptoms

As I switched to my third rheumatologist ("Dr. C") in October 2013, I stopped taking the prednisone that the second one ("Dr. B") had prescribed for me. Why would I stop taking it when I know that it's going to cause my symptoms to worsen?

Because I don't want to cover things up.

Prednisone is not a long-term solution in my mind. The long-term use of steroids is not the best for our bodies and I'd like to try to avoid it if at all possible. The reason I agreed to go on it was because it was given the same time I started the hydroxychloroquine (the second time) and the logic was "let's see if the steroid can knock your symptoms down long enough for the other meds to start working since they take 4-6 months to work." It was meant to be a blast to get things under control and then be able to treat.

I'm familiar with this method - my orthopedist did it while I was in college. He tried to take care of the symptoms (pain) in my knees to give the treatment we were trying a chance to work. It didn't work then and I ended up having surgeries on both my knees, but I understand the theory of trying it. So I agreed to go on the prednisone (and it was a low dose, which made me feel better).

That was in April 2013. I weaned off of it after about 2 months and my pain and problems came back with a vengeance (it hadn't vanished while on it but it had become more manageable). Dr. B told me to go back on it. That was in July.

I went to Dr. C for my first consult in mid-October. He went through all of my symptoms, ran extensive blood tests and X-rays and I was to come back in about 3 weeks to go over the results.

But after that initial consult with Dr. C I began to wonder just exactly how bad things are - without prednisone covering things up. If I have something covering it up, how will I know how it's progressing? How will I know if I'm getting worse, staying the same or (don't I wish!) having less severe symptoms?

So I stopped taking it. (I was on the lowest dose, so no need to wean off).

It may seem crazy (based on all the talking I've done about how constant pain every day is a drain on me mentally, physically and emotionally), that I'd want to stop taking something that helps - even if it only helps a little.

But I want to know if I'm still hurting, what type of hurting it is and how badly it hurts.

That's very different than saying I want to hurt. I don't want to hurt. I desperately want it to go away. But only if the cause of it goes away.

I don't want to be masking something that is getting

worse, or that is causing concerns for other parts of my body that is being hidden and going undetected.

Pain is one of the ways that the body says "something is going on that isn't great here and you should probably pay attention to it!" It's part of the body's warning system that you need to do something to take care of some problem. Covering up my pain and symptoms would be like turning off the smoke detectors and then getting upset that they didn't warn you that the house was burning down.

For instance, my fine motor skill issues have been present for a couple of years. However, until I went off the prednisone last month I wasn't aware of just how bad it had gotten. It has actually taken me quite by surprise how bad it is now and that's part of what scares me so much: (1) the fact that I can get that much worse that quickly and (2) the fact that I could be covering up other things that are deteriorating rapidly and I wouldn't know they were going on if I was covering them up.

Another reason that I don't like to cover things up is because I want to know they were really happening. That they weren't some figment of my imagination. Remember, this disease takes an average of 4.7 years to be diagnosed. I think a large part of that is because the symptoms are seemingly so disconnected. I would have never connected my dry eyes that I complained to my optometrist about with the fatigue that I complained to my doctor about and with the dry mouth that I never really complained to anyone about - I just dealt with it. I never would have put all those things together with the numbness and loss of fine motor control and especially not with the brain fog! The manifestations are seemingly random. However they aren't - they're all a part of this autoimmune disease.

The flip side of finally getting diagnosed is that you've seen just how random things can be related. It turns you into someone that watches like a hawk for every seemingly random symptom that you have going on. Because no one put the pieces together for so many years, now you want to make sure that all the pieces are put together and nothing else that seems random falls through the cracks. This makes you want to be aware of everything that's going on with you - if you cover things up you might miss it and not know that it's another piece of the puzzle! However, this can lead to other problems - like doctors blowing off what you say to them because they think you're a hypochondriac for bringing up every little thing to them when really you're just trying to make sure no more seemingly random pieces are left out!

I don't want the pain, fatigue, fine motor control and other problems as a constant part of my life. But I do want to be able to take an inventory of everything each day just to see where things stand.

I want to be able to flip a switch to my "actual" self and feel everything - figure out how I feel and what's going on that day - and then flip the switch to my "feel great" self and go about my day without having to deal with it all. Or maybe it could be like the updates on my computer. When there is an update available, a pop-up appears in the top corner to let me know, but I can tell it to "Try me tomorrow." I'd like my symptoms to pop-up in the morning and then have the option to say "OK, got it. Let me know tomorrow how things are going."

How bad can it really be?

My journey with this disease has often made me contemplate things I don't think I would otherwise. Some are rather random. But I guess that just shows how large of a presence in my life this has all become.

For example - is there a hierarchy to pain - does pain in one location out-rank pain in other locations? The reason this thought comes up in my mind is that people often seem to minimize my pain when I describe it as being my hands (and occasionally my toes and feet). After all, it's not my back, neck, hips or knees. I can still walk. How bad could pain in your hands really be? Our hands do seem like one of the more minor places to have pain. That is, until you realize how much you do with your hands.

It's like when you get a cut on a finger and wear a band aid on it - all of the sudden you notice how annoying it is to have that finger bandaged. It seems to get in the way of everything. My hand pain and fine motor skill issues get in the way of everything - writing, typing, cooking, shampooing my hair, crafting, driving, playing on my phone, and on and on. All of the sudden I notice just how much of an impact my hands have on my life.

So it hits you from two directions. The physical pain is bad enough, but then you add on the "frequent annoyance" factor of how often it affects your life, and it really starts to add up.

Then there are the times that I wonder if I'm somehow exaggerating what's going on with me in my own mind? Am I making a bigger deal out of the pain and fatigue than it really is? Since so many of the symptoms seem to be ramped-up versions of most peoples' lives, I wonder if my complaints are really legitimate. Everyone is tired. Everyone has aches and pains as they age. Everyone forgets things due to increasing age and busy family lives. Are my problems really any worse than any body else's?

These thoughts are often fueled by the way others (including medical professionals) react to descriptions of the pain and fatigue, the nature of an invisible disease in general, and the fact that no one has ever heard of this disease anyway. For example, when I talk about my exhaustion and someone says "I know, me too, I'm so tired from [doing whatever they've been up to lately]" or even when I first went to doctors with these symptoms in 2008 and was told it was "lifestyle stress and fatigue."

Until I remember that others are having similar struggles. Venus Williams dropped out of the US Tennis Open in August of 2011. Her fatigue and joint pain was so severe that she, a world-class athlete that was in shape and was certainly used to pushing through physical demands of training and competition, had to drop out mid-tournament. She had just been diagnosed with Sjögren's Syndrome, although she didn't make that knowledge public until after the US Open.

Venus Williams told People Magazine that "I couldn't raise my arm over my head, the racket felt like concrete. I had no feelings in my hands. They were swollen and itchy."*

I wouldn't wish this on anyone, but on some level it is reassuring to know that someone as physically sound and strong as her struggles as much as I do with the same disease. I know that she's simply another human and that her struggle is no different than the millions of others that are struggling with the same thing. There's just something about knowing that someone that surely has experienced and played through physical pain and exhaustion that any world class athlete would experience, was debilitated by the same disease that's plaguing me - it's validating. It makes me feel a little more secure in my judgment of my pain and fatigue. It makes me feel secure in the knowledge that I'm not making a mountain out of a mole-hill. It's a mountain on its own right and I, along with millions of others, am struggling over it.

---

* http://www.dailymail.co.uk/news/article-2079539/
Sjögrens-Syndrome-Venus-Williams-opens-incurable-disease.html

Symptom Creep

Many people have heard the analogy of the frog in the hot water. If you put a frog in boiling water it jumps out. But if you put a frog in room temperature water and slowly bring it up to boiling, the frog stays in.

That's what "symptom creep" does to those with chronic and degenerative diseases. If I had woken up one day 5 years ago and felt like I feel right now, I would have known there was something very wrong with me. But that's not what happened. Instead, little by little symptoms (and the severity of those symptoms) began to creep up on me.

I remember when I was first (incorrectly) diagnosed in 2011, several people would comment from time to time about how I'd never mentioned having any symptoms - that I'd never mentioned having pain or fatigue - why am I now all of the sudden diagnosed and on all these meds? Because I had been the frog in the water that was slowly warming up.

When pain or symptoms creeps up over the course of months and years, you gradually get used to it. Your "baseline of normal" shifts. Changes from day to day are minimal and you keep going, plugging along at life until you look up one day and think "How did I get to this point? I didn't always feel this way!"

This is true with all of my symptoms. I remember my dry eyes being enough of a discomfort that I talked to my optometrist about it in 2008 and she switched my brand of contacts. In order for me to have commented on it, it must have been going on for quite a while - the discomfort didn't happen over night - it built up until the point where I mentioned it to the doctor. If my eyes had felt back in 2008 like they feel now, I wouldn't have even been able to put a contact in for 5 minutes, much less wear them all day every day with only some noticeable discomfort.

Same with the loss of fine motor skills. It used to happen every once in a while - I'd shake it off as weird but not really concerning. Now it happens many times a day, sometimes for long periods of time. Again - had I experienced this "all of the sudden" I would have pushed much harder for answers when it started.

So what's the problem with "symptom creep"? Why is it something people should be aware of? Well, there's two reasons.

First, it makes it harder to be aware of disease-related symptoms and what's important to share with doctors. If we as patients don't provide them with all the possible information, it makes it harder for them to do their jobs. We're not withholding information on purpose. It's just that as our baseline of normal shifts from day-to-day or month-to-month, things may not seem "noteworthy" in the short-term comparisons we tend to focus on.

Second, one of the barriers to dealing well with these invisible diseases is being able to share and communicate with those around you about what's going on with you. They can't see the symptom creep - it's invisible. And if each day you're not dramatically different than the day before it's hard for them to understand why at some point you need to say "I've hit my limit." If you've been able to do something for a while, but then all of the sudden the cumulative effect of the creep is so great that you've hit a barrier that prevents you from continuing it, it's hard for people to realize that it's the cumulative effect of the creep and not just the difference between yesterday and today. You can "get by" for a while, but there's a breaking point - a point at which you can no longer do something. That breaking point might not look so different from the day before - but it looks very different from months or years before. But we get so lost in the everyday that we forget about the overall effect of the creep.

An analogy for this phenomenon is when my kids grow out of clothes. I know they're growing - but they don't shoot up 2 inches overnight. I see them every day and they don't really seem that different from the day before. But then all of the sudden you look at them and realize those jeans or shorts are *way* too short. They started out long, and then fit fine for a while, and then were getting short but still passable, and yet all of the sudden you look at them one day and say "no - not any more!" The kid isn't really that different from they were the last time they wore those clothes (a few days or a week before) - but they are a lot different from the first time.

At what point along the symptom creep does it become worthy enough to tell the doctor? At what point does it become too much to be able to continue to do things you've always done? And how do you explain to the doctor, friends or family why you've now all of the sudden reached a breaking point when today isn't that much different than yesterday? How do you convince them that it's valid and legitimate and severe when you haven't mentioned it before or it hasn't caused a change in your abilities up to that point? How do you get them to believe it's noteworthy or behavior change-worthy today? How do you convince a doctor that it's worthy of treatment now?

Pain Medication

There have been various times in my life when I was taking pain medication. I've taken pain meds after surgeries, following root canals, and other instances of acute pain. Real pain medication - "the good stuff" - not over-the-counter ibuprofen or acetaminophen. Over-the-counter pain medications pretty much do nothing for me...even before my current issues.

I never like taking pain meds. They tend to have a powerful effect on me (which I find funny because the over-the-counter pain meds do about as much good as eating a couple Smarties). I usually only take half the prescribed dose and I never finish the whole bottle. I don't like feeling out of it or being knocked out. I definitely don't like the ones that make me feel nauseous. And with my chronic pain now, if I took them every time I was hurting, I wouldn't be able to function.

Not that I can fully function now - but it's different. Yes, I have fatigue and brain fog that slow me down and impacts what I can spend my limited energy reserves doing, but that's different than being in a pain-medication-induced stupor. At least now I can drive my kids to school!

I did ask for a prescription one time, in the fall of 2011 while I was waiting to get through the red tape of the insurance company and specialty pharmacy to begin my first biologic injectable. They weren't the really hard stuff that incapacitates me, but it was enough to have an effect.

However, for many reasons, I just couldn't take them for long. There's just something about long-term pain medication use that sits funny with me. And it's not because I'm intellectually opposed to it. Like many of the struggles I've talked about in this book, it's a case of what I know intellectually differing from what I feel emotionally.

Intellectually I know that pain medication is there for a reason - to help us not have to experience it. But emotionally there's a lot more to it. I don't want to be someone that regularly takes pain medications long-term whether I needed it or not. There's a stigma in our society, right or wrong, about doing that. All the stories of people addicted to pain medication, taking it long after their physical injuries are healed. I'm absolutely not saying that everyone on long-term pain medication is like that - but there's certainly a social stigma about it.

So again, I managed to down-grade my pain in my own mind. Surely this pain I was experiencing couldn't possibly be long-term pain medication worthy! Surely if I was that bad then I wouldn't be able to function AT ALL. Surely my pain isn't as dire as other people that have much better justifications for using it. I have enough of a hard time trying to "justify" to others that I'm in pain at all as most people aren't used to chronic, invisible pain. How would I justify that I'm in enough pain to warrant long-term pain medication use.

And then there's the issue of "covering up" that I talked about before. Pain is your body's way of saying "Hey! Pay attention to this over here! It's not quite right and you need to

113

do something about it!" If I cover it up all the time, how will I know when it's better or worse? How will I be able to accurately judge and communicate my pain level (when I clearly have such issues doing that anyway - even without the added layer of pain medication covering it up)?

But what if it gets to the point where we know what's causing the pain, we know why it's there but there's just nothing that we can do to stop it? What if I try all of the treatments for my disease out there and nothing works to relieve my symptoms? Then is it OK to cover it up - knowing it's still there but not needing it to be an alarm-system for my body any longer?

I never had these emotional issues taking pain medication for short-term pain. It was clearly justified after a surgery or injury. The doctors only prescribed it for a short time - usually with no refills, and I know that whatever healing needs to happen will be over shortly and I'll be able to be off it. I don't have all the hang-ups using it short-term that I seem to have long-term.

For now I'm able to moderately function in my life without it. It makes me crabby, not much fun to be around and drained from dealing with the pain all the time. For now at least, that's the lesser of two evils when comparing my current state to how I would be on long-term pain medications. But what happens if or when that's no longer the case?

What happens when the pain gets to a point where it's no longer the lesser of two evils to suffer through it? At what point does the need for palliative care outweigh the concerns for long-term pain medication use? What do I do at that point? Will I be able to realize that I'm at the point where being on pain medications is better for myself and those around me than not being on them? Will the "symptom creep" be so slow that I don't realize I'm at that point? And even if I'm able to recognize that point, will the doctors? Will they understand what this is like to go through? Will I get the palliative care that I need or will I be labeled as a drug seeker?

Why I Hate Glasses

I've talked about what I consider my scariest symptom to date - my loss of fine motor skills. Now I'll talk about something that's not as severe as that…and if I step back and look at it, it even makes me laugh at how I complain about it when I have far worse things going on. But never-the-less, it's an issue and I'm going to vent about it!

I started wearing contacts in 8th grade. I convinced my parents to get them for me because I was a cheerleader and I couldn't see the score (or anything else, really) while I was cheering. It wasn't like it is now - with the throw-away kind. They were expensive, and if they were lost or torn you didn't just open up a new package from the box. You had one pair and that was it. I distinctly remember being made to empty out the trap under the sink into a metal pan and sift through the gunk to rescue a contact that I'd let go down the sink drain as a teenager. Just the thought of that makes me gag, even now!

I remember when I first got them, I walked around saying "You people actually see this stuff…without glasses or contacts?" I truly had no idea that this was the way people were supposed to see!

My first pair of glasses was in second grade (remarkably

the exact same age both of my children began wearing them). They were pretty sweet (insert sarcasm here!). Rose-tinted lenses that were huge (and not in the trendy-over-sized-sun-glasses way, but rather in the it-was-the-80's-way) with my initials in the corner with stickers! I'm not sure exactly when I quit wearing glasses but they disappeared from school pictures somewhere around 4th grade, so I'm thinking they didn't last very long. Now years later I think I know why. Because I hate them! But my eyes gradually got worse between the revolt from glasses and the arrival of contacts.

Currently I can see enough that, if in an emergency I had to be able to function, I could do so. I'm not as bad as my son who can't even see the giant "E" at the top of the chart without his corrective lenses, but I can't see details for anything about a foot and a half away from my face without corrective lenses. So constant corrective lenses are necessary for pretty much everything in my life except for laying in bed reading with the Kindle about 8 inches from my face.

In April 2013, I was told by the ophthalmologist that I could not wear contacts. I, of course, starting asking if I could "just wear them" for various things, like to dance or for photography. He said absolutely not - that I was doing damage to my eyes by wearing them because of the chronic dry eyes due to my Sjögren's. I asked if I could have Lasik and he said - and I'm literally quoting him, word for word here, "Oh, hell no!" He said that maybe, after my eyes had begun to recover, that maybe I could begin to work up a tolerance for wearing contacts for brief periods of time, but that I need to be prepared to never wear them again. And now that it's been a while since that conversation I know this ban on contacts is likely permanent – the issues are not getting better.

My point to this story is that doctors need to be more aware of when something may seem inconsequential to them but yet have major impact on their patient's lives. It may seem very easy for him to say "don't wear contacts - just wear glasses." But for the patient it may be much more important than that.

I know some people choose glasses over contacts - my brother, in fact, chooses glasses because the thought of poking his eye gives him the heebie-jeebies. Then again, his vision isn't nearly as bad as mine, as evidenced when he and my kids began a "glasses swap" when we went to visit him last year - he and my daughter are about the same, mine are significantly worse and my son's are off the charts worse. He can still do things without them (like swimming) and get by relatively easily. Some people are completely OK with wearing them everyday even if they can't see well enough to manage without them, and that's great for them.

But for me it's a loss of the choice. I don't get to choose glasses because I want to, I'm told I have to have them because I have no other choice. I can't have surgery. I can't use overnight corneal reshaping like my son does now. I can't wear contacts just for various activities. I have no choice. This stupid disease has taken away so much and now it's taking this away, too.

Yes, I know there are worse things in my life, and much worse things in others' lives, than taking away my choice of corrective lenses. But it's symbolic. It's symbolic of how it's affecting every little aspect of my life. And there's nothing I can do about it.

So here are all the reasons that I hate wearing glasses, most of which I never even considered before I had to wear them every day. After all, it's been since 3rd or 4th grade since

I've worn them daily.

1. I can't see with them off to put make-up on, but I have to have them off to put the make-up on.
2. They cover up that make-up that I just put on, so you know what...let's just skip the make-up all together.
3. They fog up when I go from an air conditioned house or car to the Kansas summer humidity.
4. They fog up when I open the oven door.
5. They fog up when I pour something hot into the strainer. Have you ever been in the middle of pouring hot, boiling liquid and suddenly not been able to see. Food has ended up missing the strainer and landing in the sink because of this. Boiling water has been spilled on me because of this. Not fun.
6. They fog up when I open the dishwasher.
7. I get zits under the nose piece and that really hurts.
8. I can't lay on my side on the couch and watch TV.
9. I can't see when I swim - in fact I never went under the water this entire summer because I can't stand to not be able to see - so I spent the last two summers in the pool keeping my head above water.
10. I have to have a second set of glasses as prescription sunglasses. Not only does this cost more money, but then I do dumb things like get out of the car and go into a store only to realize I still have my sunglasses on and have to turn back around and go back to the car and get my regular glasses. I can't do the transitions lenses because I can't have the tinting for photography (see below). I don't like the clip-on things...and frankly, I'd lose them...or break them...I know myself too well for that.
11. It's hard to be a photographer with them - I don't like having my glasses between me and my camera (I use the viewfinder, not a digital screen to compose my shots). If I wear sun-

glasses outside (at my kids' sporting events or just anywhere outside) and want to take picture then I have to flip back and forth between my sunglasses and regular glasses, or I have to flip my sunglasses up on top of my head to check exposure - but then I can't see!

12. They slip when they get sweaty.

13. I can't dance with them on. It was a few months before the dance show I was a part of in 2013 when this all came about. I couldn't see in dance class (let alone have any reliable balance) with them off, but if I had them on they went flying off constantly.

14. Likewise, I can't exercise in general with them on without them constantly slipping, shifting and causing my vision to do funny things as they do so.

15. I get sore spots behind my ears.

16. I have to take them off to rub my face or eyes.

17. It's irritating to pull up a ponytail or get your hair cut or colored and have to have them off the whole time.

18. I have to turn my head to be able to see - I can't just shift my eyes up, down, left or right...I actually have to turn my head.

19. I have to push them up all the time.

20. I can't hug my husband without them being pushed into the side of my face (similar to laying on my side)

21. I'm sure there's more...I curse them in my head on a regular basis...that's just all I can think of right now.

Brain Fog

My "thing" has always been that I'm smart. I was never really athletic. I danced, but once college was over, other than the occasional classes for recreation, I stopped dancing and performing. I'm mildly creative, but not in a way that is as much a part of "who I am" like my "smarts."

I'm smart. I graduated high school with the max amount of college credits that I could (30); got a full-ride to a private, liberal-arts undergraduate college to study chemistry; began publishing research and education articles in peer-reviewed journals during my first year of teaching (because I wanted to - not because it was tied to any sort of graduate degree…I hadn't even started my masters at that point); wrote a high-school chemistry textbook; received regional and national awards for my teaching; earned a PhD (paid for through academic fellowships I earned by my "smarts").

I have other components to my self-identity (mother, wife, friend, creative, etc.) but my brain, academic and career success is a major part of it. I'm proud of it.

I am an educator. I taught high school chemistry for 10 years. Even now that I'm no longer in the classroom I'm still an educator. I work with science graduate students and high school teachers as they partner to bring the grad student's research into the science classroom - including leading the weekly graduate student seminar course and parts of the annual summer institute they attend. I still lead workshops for teachers; I still present at national conferences; I continue to be in front of groups of people teaching and leading discussions. I mention this part because I'm very comfortable talking in front of groups of all sizes - I'm used to it.

About two years ago I noticed that something wasn't the same when I was teaching or leading classes and workshops. I couldn't find words that I wanted to use. And not in the occasional way that everyone experiences from time to time. But in a frequent way. A way that was causing me to not be able to express the thoughts in my head. A way that was happening so often that I realized something was going on with me.

I'd find myself part-way through a thought while talking to the group and not be able to finish it, not be able to find the words I needed. They were there in my mind but somehow just outside of my grasp.

This happened often enough that I was noticing it and wondering what the heck was going on with me. I wasn't imagining it, it happened frequently and I'm way too young for it to be due to aging.

At some point after this had been going on for a while I learned about brain fog. Brain fog is associated with many autoimmune disease like Sjögren's, MS or Lupus. In some instances, people with "brain fog" have been seen to have inflammation in areas of blood vessels inside the brain. Autoimmune diseases can cause inflammation everywhere, causing all kinds of havoc: moisture-producing glands = tears and saliva issues;

blood vessels around nerves = neuropathy; blood vessels in brain = brain fog.

> "What is Brain Fog? Brain Fog is a lay term to describe fluctuating mild memory loss that is inappropriate for a person's age. It may include forgetfulness, spaciness, confusion, decreased ability to pay attention, an inability to focus, and difficulty in processing information. Remember that gradual cognitive decline from early adulthood is a fact of life. Brain Fog can occur in Sjögren's syndrome (SS), but other factors might cause these symptoms and should be considered by you and your doctor." *

I first read about "brain fog" when I was given a "possible" diagnosis of Lupus in April 2013 and began to research it. Brian fog is common in Lupus and appeared in information about Lupus frequently (as opposed to the research I'd been doing on RA for a couple of years when that had been my diagnosis - I'd never run across it in that information).

By the time I began to read about it, it had already been happening for quite a while. Long enough that I'd noticed it already and was wondering what was going on with me. So I know it wasn't a case of developing symptoms after I learn about their possibility. With physical symptoms I don't worry so much about developing them after I've learned about them - they're physical. But with this mental one I'm glad I developed and noticed it before I learned about it…I don't want to make myself believe that I'm "imagining it" simply because I learned it was a possibility.

Nope…this really is happening to me.

---

* http://www.Sjögren's.org/files/brochures/brain_fog.pdf

And what makes this all the harder to deal with in the medical world is that it could be caused by physical manifestations - inflammation of blood vessels in the brain, but it can also be caused by the other symptoms of the disease. I'm fatigued. I'm stressed. I'm dealing with a lot and trying to still maintain as normal of a life as possible. Just like when they say kids dealing with poverty and lack of enough to eat means they aren't able to learn as well when they go to school hungry - people going through life fatigued, stressed, and plagued with a variety of chronic symptoms are less likely to function as they did prior to all of these issues.

Who knows if the brain fog I'm experiencing is a physical manifestation of my disease or if it's related to the other symptoms, or some combination of the two, but it's there and it's a part of my daily struggle.

I've always been one of the most efficient people I know. At one point I had a 4 year-old, a 2 year-old, taught high school full time, was in grad school working towards my PhD and was finishing the publishing process for that chemistry textbook. I juggled it all, rarely forgot anything that I needed to do, and got it all done.

Now I can't even remember to do the most simple things. I use my technology to try to keep myself on track - a calendar and to-do list software that syncs to all 3 computers, my iPhone and my iPad. I have it with me everywhere and I still forget stuff far to frequently for my happiness! And that's even with a "stripped-down" life of responsibilities since I simply can't juggle as much as I used to handle.

So then I start to look at the "tips for living with Brain

Fog" that places like the Sjögren's Foundation put out there…

The most prevalent tip is "Train your brain…if you don't use it, you lose it!" Ummm…I'm pretty sure I'm using my brain enough. I have a "thinking" job, I have "thinking" side-jobs (educational author and presenter) and I even have "thinking" hobbies (like programming apps for the fun of it and writing). I use my brain plenty, thank you…and it's not helping!

The second tip that makes me outright laugh is "To help symptoms of 'brain fog,' minimize stress and anxiety. Take breaks throughout the day and learn relaxation exercises and practice them at regular intervals."

Seriously? The "brain fog" is one of the things causing me stress and anxiety - along with every other aspect of living with this disease. And taking breaks throughout the day adds to the stress and anxiety because I just sit there and think about all of the things I *should* be doing instead of taking that break! (And let's not forget the guilt for someone with chronic illness and fatigue that taking breaks brings…adding even more anxiety!)

And finally…"Letting yourself laugh and talk about your feelings will help reduce stress and anxiety, which contribute to fatigue and 'brain fog' in Sjögren's."

I have a hard time feeling like people really believe the physical symptoms I've having from this invisible disease…how in the heck am I'm going to convince anyone that I'm having cognitive symptoms? "Let yourself laugh and talk about your feelings"? Maybe some day I'll be able to laugh about it. But not now. Not yet. And these tips and advice don't help with the right now.

I can barely talk about this stuff with my husband (in fact I don't think I've talked about my brain fog symptoms at all), let alone laugh and talk about it with everyone around. I can only write about it here because (1) I'm forcing myself to do it as a way of dealing with it and (2) even though I know my friends and family can read this, it's still feels way more "anonymous" than sitting down with someone face-to-face and trying to explain my "brain fog," an act I fear would be met with either "girl, we're all running around forgetting stuff because we're so busy" or "you're just imagining it."

This is more than "busy with children and all that is going on in life and forgetting things." I experienced that for years. This is "I can't think of words to say that I should be able to say." This is "I can't express my thoughts - I can feel them there, just below the surface but I can't grasp onto them, I can't get them to the surface to get them out."

And for someone that has spent many, many years of her life with "smart girl" being a large part of her self-identity, it's disheartening, it's discouraging, it's feeling like this stupid disease is reaching into every part of my being and pulling pieces away. Nothing is safe from it…at least that's how it makes me feel.

It's in the Genes

Autoimmune diseases are very poorly understood. Most information seems to indicate that they are the result of a complex interaction between genetics and environment. Perhaps some people are predisposed to them based on genetics and they're "kick-started" by an environmental factor - maybe a virus or cold that gets the immune system going and then it goes haywire from there.

In October 2013, a study was released indicating six genes have been found to be associated with Sjögren's*. This is a huge step forward in the ability to someday understand this disease.

I have zero doubt that I have the genes they found. And the reason why I'm convinced of that is because my maternal grandmother had Sjögren's, although she was never diagnosed.

My Mamaw died in late 2010. She can't be diagnosed now, but I'm certain this is what plagued her for many years. She was the same as me.

First, she always had a "through the roof sed rate"

---

* http://www.sciencedaily.com/releases/2013/10/131006142446.htm

(as one of my rheumatologists phrased it). Sed rate is a very non-specific way of telling that there is inflammation in the body. My mom says they always told Mamaw that it was high but could never find a reason for it.

Second, she had chronic dry eyes and mouth - she complained of it often. Although those are by far not the only symptoms of Sjögren's, they are a hallmark.

Third, fatigue and joint pain. Mom says she complained of these things for many years as well.

Both of my parents remember her struggling with these issues for most of their adult lives. She'd go to doctors and they'd write her off or giver a B-12 shot and send her on her way.

Fourth, we're genetically related. I actually look quite a lot like her. I'd been told that often when I was little but had a hard time comparing my little girl face to her grandma face. When I was older and saw pictures of her from when she was younger, I began to see it. And if I got genes from her that are visible, there's no reason not to think that we both suffer from the same symptoms and that those are genetically linked as well. My aunt, Mamaw's daughter, is also struggling with Sjögren's. She's on of those 2 million people that are sero-negative (she doesn't have the antibodies showing up in her blood-work that indicate Sjögren's) and is fighting for diagnosis through the VA system. So now there's three generations of Sjögren's in our family.

I'm so very sorry that she suffered while doctors wrote off her symptoms or just ignored them. I'm very sorry that she never learned the name of what was wrong with her and to feel that little bit of satisfaction that comes with knowing it's not "all in your head."

But I know she loved me dearly and I know that she's somewhere, very happy right now that I'm making progress with it and fighting to find treatments that work for me.

I also know, without even the slightest doubt, that wherever she is, she's saying in her southern drawl "I *told* them something wasn't right!" now that she's seeing that it is a "real" thing that wasn't "in her head!" Mamaw had a widely known way of letting people know when she was right all along, and it always began with "I *told* them..." And anyone that knew her can hear in his or her head exactly how she said that phrase!

So in honor of Mamaw, each time throughout this long and winding autoimmune disease process that I'm right about something and have to push doctors to get there, I'll be saying "I *told* them" in my head!

How long are you allowed to be sad, angry and upset with chronic illness?

When I pose the question of "How long are you allowed to be sad, angry and upset with chronic illness?" I'm not talking about how long can the periods of sadness last. I know that it cannot be indefinite. I have to pick myself up and move on. I have to be sad, angry or upset in order to process what's going on with me and, when that's done, then I can move on to the next step. We have to let ourselves feel and process our emotions in order to deal with them, but then we have to move on to the logic and functioning of life. I can't check out of everything indefinitely - I have responsibilities and a life to lead.

Instead, I'm talking about how long can those periods occur? How long after your diagnosis are you allowed to have those periods? How long until someone says (or you think it in your own head) "You've been diagnosed for x years - it's time to move on and get over it (and not have those periods - no matter how short or long - anymore)"?

When you have acute injuries or illness, there's a natural progression to your feelings about the injury or illness. There's a beginning and there's an end. It doesn't last forever and you move on. You may have feelings of anger or sadness, but when the injury or illness has run its course, you can move on.

With chronic illnesses, it's never run its course. You never really get to move on.

This is something that I struggle with a lot. It appears to be a never-ending cycle. The phases may last hours, days, weeks or months, but they seem to keep going in the cycle.

It begins with sadness and anger - why do I have to deal with this? Why do I have to have my life turned upside down like this? Why can't I effectively communicate what's really going on with me? Why don't other people understand that it's constant, despite the fact that it's invisible?

And then it turns to guilt and shame. There are always people worse off than I am. There are always people with troubles greater than mine. I can't be making withdrawals from the relationship banks to help me deal with my issues without making deposits as well. This phase causes me to push it down - to try to ignore it and carry on like normal, but that can't be sustained. It can't last very long before the pain, fatigue, mental and emotional stress gets to be too much and I break down.

Then comes the sadness and anger again. Why should I have to hide what's going on with me (even if it's my own guilt and shame making me feel like I have to hide it and nothing anybody else says or does to make me feel that way)? Why should I have to pretend to be fine and go about my life when I'm not? Don't I have a right to express what's going on with me and to live within my limits?

And it cycles back around to the guilt and shame. I can't always feel bad for myself. Who am I to expect special treatment - even if it's just having my husband do more than his fair share around the house because I'm too tired or hurting to do my share? After all that others have done for me to help me reach my goals and accomplish the many things in my life, how can I retreat and give those parts of my life up and not reach my potential?

How do I balance my own expectations for myself, others' expectations for me and my physical and emotional limits? How can I remind others of those physical and emotional limits without feeling like I'm a constant whiner? How can I deal with others assuming I should be doing more because they forget or aren't fully aware - instead of snapping at them because I'm tired of having to defend myself when I can't do things?

How do I accept it and move on when just when I think I've reached the point of being able to do that another symptom occurs? Or doctors run additional tests to check for an overlap in diagnoses? Or things substantially worsen?

There's so much advice out there (online, in books, and from well-meaning people) to get on with your life, not let your disease define you, not let it change who you are and what you do. How can you do those things when you never know when fatigue will hit, when you're not sure if you'll be able to do things you've made plans to do? How can you not let it change things when you never know if tomorrow's pain will be bad enough to cause you to cancel your plans? How can you not let it define you, when you physically can't do the things that used to be such a big part of your identity and self-concept (like teach all day, hold the heavy SLR camera and lens for long periods of time photographing, sew or do other crafting, etc.)?

How can I redefine myself to take into account all of these realities of my life in a way that doesn't make me feel like less than I was or less than I should be? How can I help others to understand my re-defined self without feeling immense guilt or feeling like I'm letting others down, or having to deal with issues of others thinking I've changed, accusing me of not pulling my weight or that I'm stuck-up or something else? Maybe I'll have the answers to these questions one day, but after years of asking the questions I don't have the answers yet.

Isolation

I think most people just want to be left alone when they don't feel good. When we have the flu, a killer headache, a fever or other type of "I don't feel good" ailment, most of us just want to be left alone. A "don't talk to me, don't ask me talk to you, I don't care about idle chit-chat, and don't ask me where your [whatever object you can't find that I'm sure is right in front of your face but because you're a 11 year-old boy, you're incapable of seeing it for yourself] is" kind of "leave me alone" feeling.

That works fine in the short term. You hide in your room, snuggle under a blanket, watch some mindless TV and in a few days you feel better. Others generally understand this process, except the occasional child that insist that you are the only person on the planet that can solve their particular problem at that particular moment...they don't quite get the "leave me alone" concept - but otherwise, most people get it. We tend to cut each other slack when a sick person seems distant or withdrawn.

But what happens when that "I don't feel good" period lasts years?

I have times that aren't as bad as others, but there are large chunks of times - weeks and months at a time - when it's a struggle to not want to just be left alone. I don't feel like making much of an effort. I don't feel like talking. Even if I was to talk, what's on my mind is what's going on with me and I completely understand that other people have other things going on in their lives and no one wants to talk about what's going on in mine all the time.

So combine the "I just want to be left alone" phenomenon with the understanding that no one wants to hear about what's going on with me all the time and add that together with the struggles of a disease being invisible that I've talked about earlier, and what you end up with is isolation.

It's like life is on pause for me, yet it's moving on for everyone else and leaving me behind. I don't blame anyone. Relationships are two way streets and I know I haven't held up my end. I haven't shown as much interest as I should (or want to) in others and what's going on in their lives. I haven't reached out to others and invited them places or to do things. I haven't hung out with friends like I used to. I completely understand that this isolation was my own doing. On some level it's easier to be left alone - in a strange way it's what I want: to be left alone and not have to keep up appearances or pretend like everything is fine when I'm physically hurting or frustrated or anxious about what's going on (which takes energy that I'm trying to conserve).

It's very easy to say things like "you can't let it stop your life" and "you have to keep on going" and "just ignore it and live your life." And I probably would have thought those things before this all happened. But after years of trying one medicine after another, musical diagnoses and searching for the "right" doctor — the entire time dealing with chronic pain, fatigue, brain fog and fine motor skill issues - it's very, very hard to do those things on a daily basis.

I feel like I haven't been "normal" in years. Yes, I can act "normal" - but not for very long. I can do it for a short period of time, but not consistently, day in and day out for almost 3 years.

I feel like I can't show how I'm really feeling and what I'm really thinking - everyone would get tired of it, of hearing me whine, of hearing about my problems when they have their own.

So what's the problem with the isolation? If I want to be left alone and can't keep up the appearance of "being normal," then why am I now unhappy with feeling isolated? Because I miss myself and part of what I miss about myself is my relationships with others. I miss how I was always willing to do things for others. I miss how close I felt to friends and my husband. I miss being invited places. I miss feeling like I had a social life. Instead I feel very distant and superficial. I recognize it, I understand how it happened, I want to go back to normal...but yet I just can't do it perpetually...not yet. And I'm afraid that if I am ever ready and able that everyone will have moved on in the meantime.

But you did that, why can't you do this?

In the summer of 2012 my husband, kids and I went on a vacation to Florida. After visiting with my grandpa and aunt for a night, we went to Cocoa Beach for a day and played on the beach (my parents actually used to live there...although I love having them close on a daily basis now that live by me, I do miss my free vacation spot that I used to have access to...it definitely beat staying in a hotel!)

The next day we went to Kennedy Space Center. If you've never been, it's a phenomenally cool place (although it is rather pricey!) My son was 10 and was a great age to visit there. We spent the day and had a great time. We stopped for dinner before we headed back inland. While at dinner, my son convinced me to go back out to the beach for just a little bit before heading to central Florida for the night (we had plans to go to Sea World and Aquatica for the next two days). I'm completely convinced that I'm made to live on a beach...so it doesn't take a whole lot of effort to get me to go back for a bit.

As we were leaving the restaurant, I was walking and rolled my ankle. Not just a little roll - an "I heard a very loud pop-pop and now can't get up" roll! And I even had tennis shoes on (I usually live in flip flops, but I'd worn tennis shoes for the walking at Kennedy that day)! And I was literally just walking! I've danced for 20+ years of my life (and in fact was taking contemporary dance class that summer as I have off-and-on over the years) and yet I roll my ankle horribly bad simply walking to the car from the restaurant.

My husband drove us across the street to the drug store and got some instant ice packs. I couldn't stand to disappoint my kiddos that were planning on time at the beach, so we went ahead and headed to the beach - me with an ice pack on my ankle and barely able to walk. Just in case you think I might be exaggerating it just a smidge, here's what it looked like the

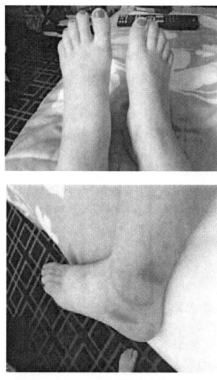

morning after it happened.

The next day we went to Sea World and I took one for the team and limped all over Sea World. The day after that, we went to Aquatica (Sea World's water park) and yep, I sucked it up through that, too. It was a really good thing that we did Sea World first because after walking around there for the day I couldn't get tennis shoes on the day we went to Aquatica...which worked well because we all just wore flip flops and then went barefoot! The following day we traveled back home - airports and airplanes (wearing flip flops - couldn't get that tennis shoe back on!). Painful, all of it!

So what does this story have to do with a book on auto-immune disease, chronic pain & chronic fatigue? I spent those two days at amusement parks, and a third day going through a major airport, and when I got home that night and the next day, all I wanted to do was sit on the couch and do nothing. I didn't want to go up and down stairs. I didn't want to run around and find whatever it is my kids were looking for. I didn't want to stand and cook. I didn't want to do anything that required me to move or put weight on that ankle. But the problem was that I had spent 3 days walking around on it (despite my mother and everyone else back home seeing pictures on Facebook telling me to go to an ER and stay off of it for the remainder of the vacation). My family got used to me being able to walk around and do things and they didn't really understand why I couldn't continue to do that once we'd gotten home.

Chronic pain and fatigue is often the same. People see you suck it up and function for specific events or short periods of time and then get frustrated when you can't do it afterwards. Just because I managed to limp through Florida in order to not be stuck sitting in a hotel room while my family enjoyed their vacation didn't mean that my pain and injury was any less severe. In fact, I more than likely did more damage to my ankle and increased the time it took to heal by doing that - short term gain (fun with my family) for long term loss (longer healing time).

In my head, I knew what my plan was - suck it up and get through the vacation and then sit with it up and rest it until it healed when I got home. The problem was that everyone else saw the first part of that plan in action and assumed I therefore didn't need the second part! And that was with a very visible injury (bruised, swollen, nasty looking ankle sitting up on the ottoman). It's even more frustrating when the recovery period is for invisible struggles because those around me can't just look at me and visibly see why I need to recover!

When I make choices about what I'm going to spend energy on, when I'm going to suck it up and put my happy face on, it sometimes backfires on me because then I frustrate those around me when I can't maintain it. "Well if you could do it for that [day, event, person, group] then why can't you do it now?" Everyone makes choices in what they spend their time and energy on in life, but those of us with chronic pain and chronic fatigue have less energy to start with - our choices must be that much more selective.

And our recovery time is much longer than other people experience. Just like I had to wait longer for my ankle to heal because I'd walked on it for those three days, each time I wear myself out I have to wait longer to bounce back. I led a workshop for teachers at a local university recently. I was so physically worn-out from that experience that it took me a full 2 days to recover from it. I taught a group for 6 hours and it took me 2 days to recover. And those two days were not much of a picnic for those around me as I exhibited my cranky self during that recovery time.

Parenting

When I was first diagnosed with an with autoimmune disease, my children were 5 and 7 years old. I want my kids to be kids as long as possible. They shouldn't have to be concerned with adult things like bills, work, stress, illnesses and so on. So for a long time I didn't tell my kids anything. Nothing at all.

But there's a problem with that and I didn't realize it at first. My condition, the number of doctor's appointments and the side-effects of the meds I was on impacted their lives.

The symptom that showed up first was fatigue. Fatigue is a major factor in my life now. Just as with my pain - some days are better than others - but it's a major factor nonetheless. It's hard to hide from the kids. It causes me to experience a great amount of guilt.

Mommy's too tired. Mommy needs to rest. Mommy can't run around and do all the things with you that she wishes she could.

These are my realities. And it breaks my heart.

I think every good parent worries that they aren't doing

absolutely everything right - none of us are perfect, none of us can do everything and anyone that is a contentious parent would worry about that at some level. Not worry about it to the point of obsession, but be enough concerned about it that we always try to do our best.

So there's the normal amount of "am I the best parent I could be?" parent guilt and worry. And then there's the "this invisible disease that you guys don't really understand, or for that matter don't even know about, is causing me to be far less physically active with my children, not to mention often makes me in a bad mood." I have a huge fear that my kids will look back on their childhood and feel like their mom was lazy or didn't play with them.

My husband was taking the kids somewhere and texted me that they were cracking him up. He said "These kids are hilarious." One the one hand, this warms my heart incredibly. That their step-dad has so whole-heartedly taken these kids a part of his life makes me very happy. But on the other hand this made me very sad. I want to have fewer times of stress, fatigue, pain and general in-a-bad-mood so I can enjoy their hilarity more. I want to be able to just enjoy their personalities and their company more. It's not that I don't at all - it's just that I want more. I want less time of having to deal with all that I'm going through and more time to be the mom I want to be.

And then there was the medicine. Some medicines that I tried had horrible side-effects. One made me feel like a zombie…I didn't just have periods of fatigue, it was non-stop. Some of the medicines were self-injectables and my children were aware that I was giving myself shots. And depending on which set of meds I'm on at any giving moment, there are often many different medicine bottles on my bathroom counter. Far more than the average 36-year-old mom.

There are also the doctor appointments and blood work. I tried to schedule my appointments for when they were in school, but during the summer they'd know about them and occasionally they came with me to get blood drawn for labs. They were aware that I was going to doctors more than most people.

So I finally realized that it would better to be more upfront about it all. Hiding things from them to "protect them" just made is so that they didn't have a clue why things were changing. And although I don't want my fatigue or pain to be an excuse for not being as active with my kids as I'd like, I would like my kids to realize that it's not because I'm lazy, don't want to or don't care.

But how much is the right amount? How much do I share? How much can they understand without scaring them or making them worry? These are not easy questions.

Mostly I refer to it as "mommy's health issues." The kids know that I have health stuff going on that causes pain and fatigue, makes me so that I can't wear contacts and that causes me to go to doctors and try to figure out which meds will work for me. But I haven't addressed the "autoimmune" aspect yet. We haven't talked about the fact that it's permanent…there is no cure. And we haven't talked about that fact that autoimmune diseases can be degenerative and I may get worse over time. They have said "I hope I don't have those issues, too," to which I respond "me, too!" after which I say a quick prayer that they don't. Especially with how autoimmune disease has a genetic link…I pray that the genes aren't triggered in their bodies someday.

For now that's where we're at. I don't know if it's enough, too much or about right. But mostly I'm just cranky that this is one more stress and concern in my life caused by the fact that my body is attacking itself. Stupid diseases.

Parenting - Part 2

I wrote the previous chapter on parenting a year before this one (more about why it took me a year to finish this book later!) Kids change a lot in a year. So here's a more recent example of parenting with chronic illness.

Slowly over the last year they've learned more about it. They know that it's the part of my body that usually fights the germs and illnesses but that it's fighting my own parts instead. They know it causes pain, dry symptoms, fatigue. They know that the medicine I'm on isn't working and that it's been frustrating. I'm honest with them when they ask me to do something - like those crazy loom band bracelets that thank goodness we're "over" in my household - that I just can't do because of hand pain or dexterity.

They know I'm frustrated with my current (actually past, as I'm not going back to him) doctor and that I have an appointment in Philadelphia in December 2014 (after my previous experience with Dr. C causing me to write him that letter!) to see a Sjögren's specialist.

Last night my daughter asked if there was a cure for my disease. When I answered "no," she asked if it had an effect on how long people lived. I said that the disease itself doesn't really, but that people with this disease often get other disease that do have an effect on how long they live (which is true – Sjögren's patients have increased risk of lymphoma and lung diseases, etc.). She then asked if I had any of those things as well and I was happy to answer "no, not right now." This is a very difficult discussion to have with your 9 year old daughter that shouldn't have to worry about these things at all at her age! They know that I had a horrible headache every day for two months in late summer/early fall of 2014 and were happy with me when it "broke" (the headache "breaking" feels just like a fever when it breaks – relief).

Both of my children are bright and caring people and show genuine concern when I do let them know that I'm having a particularly hard day (it has to be a really hard day before that happens - I'm still not good at sharing my pain/fatigue levels on medium or medium-hard days yet - I still tend to hide that from people). My son has always been especially empathetic, even from a very young age - very tenderhearted and concerned about others. He left his childhood Pooh Bear stuffed animal that he used to use to comfort himself when he was little (that these days is usually flung to the corner of his bedroom - too old to acknowledge it on a regular basis but not ready to get rid of it or pack it away in the basement) on my bed one day to help me feel better when I came home again with a headache. But even with such kind and understanding kids, I still have very active concerns that they are going to look back on their childhood later in life and think that I wasn't there for them enough - not active enough, resting too much, etc.

So a few weeks ago (at the height of my chronic head-aches), I was at the kids' school before their school carnival setting up the ticket-sales booth I was working at. I ran into the main office to ask for some pens and the principal mentioned that she was in my son's classroom (6th grade) the day before and that he was sharing about me. I was surprised and asked what he was sharing about. She said they were talking about people that "lived above the line" (the phrase that ties in with their character education and behavior code, etc.) and about people in their lives that were brave and that he talked about me and how I've had a hard couple of years. He talked about how every time we think one thing is getting better or under control something else starts to happen and that we just can't get things better. He shared about how I've done all that I do to take care of the kids and be supportive of them even though I've had a really hard couple of years.

On the one hand that's completely heartbreaking to me to know that my sweet children have to deal with chronic illness in their lives. (I just realized that this chapter is making them sound a little angelic. Don't get me wrong - they're still kids that are normal kids...they frustrate the heck out of me at bedtime, pick on each other when they get bored, drive me batty in a million small ways like kids everywhere do to all mothers! But they have good hearts and I try to frequently let them know that I'm proud of the people they are - of the hearts they have. They're kind and caring).

To know that it's impacting them to the point that my son (whom has just as hard of time verbally voicing his feelings and concerns as I do - I write in blog posts to get my feelings out, he writes me notes when he has something he needs to express to me) would share it with his class and teacher is gut wrenching. To know that he's that aware of it when he should be carefree (or at least his cares should be about childhood things - not illnesses!) is just wrong.

But a part of me finds it reassuring. He talked about me

while they were sharing about people that "live above the line." He shared this information when discussing people that are brave in their everyday lives. Maybe I am managing to make my kids feel loved and supported despite my fears of this illness causing me to not be there for them like I'd like to be. I sincerely hope so, because other than having them grow up safe and healthy, that is probably my number one wish for my kids.

Maintaining "Me"

I've come to the realization that lately my life contains a lot of "lesser of two evils" decisions. I'm faced with a lot of choices where neither outcome is exactly pleasant. I know that I'm an adult and not everything is rainbows and unicorns, and as an adult we're often making choices that aren't always pleasant. But it just seems like things are on a whole new playing field when dealing with chronic illness.

For example, I can't do everything I used to. Between pain and fatigue, I just can't. So what do I skip or give up?

The hobbies or interests I had? While they aren't strictly necessary to the running of my family or doing my job I do believe they are important to my self-concept and happiness, which does impact my family and work. I think everyone should have something they do just for them - that's not about their children or significant other, but something that's just for their soul. I've already given up mine, for the most part, because I don't the energy, or they physically hurt.

Or tasks around the house? I do very little around the house and my poor husband has been picking up the slack for me, but that doesn't sit well with me...I hate being "that wife."

Or do I give up fun things with my kids? I already don't have the energy to physically play with them like I used to...I hate telling them I'm too tired to do something.

Do I give up my long-term career goals because I can't put in the effort to maintain the work along the way that is necessary to reach them? I've worked so hard for so long and still have contributions to make - the thought of walking away from it all hurts.

No matter what I choose to give up in order to be able to do the other things, I'm losing something. I know that no one can do everything - we all make choices in where we put our time, energy and focus...but these are things that I used to be able to do...things that I really believe that if I wasn't dealing with this disease that I'd be able to continue to do.

One of the most common pieces of advice I find when looking for help is to stay active, or try to continue to do the things that bring you happiness. I've tried to do that with two areas - dance and photography.

With the exception of about five years when I had babies or toddlers at home, dance has been a part of my life since I was 3. I danced at studios and on school teams growing up and continued ballet class and performances throughout college. During my first few years of teaching high school I coached high school dance teams. I took a break while having my kids, but even after that I would occasionally take class at the studio where my daughter danced.

It's my happy place. It clears my mind, it makes me feel good, it gives me a way to express myself, and I just in general feel like myself. During 2012-2013, I decided to take class throughout the entire academic year instead of just dropping in during the summer session. I joined the high school contemporary class one night a week at the studio.

No matter how much I loved it, there were still many times that I just didn't want to go. The fatigue would be too much, or I would just be physically hurting and couldn't do things in class. With very few exceptions, I made it to class. And most of those exceptions where due to things my kids had going on - school music programs and things like that. At first it was a matter of principle - I was going to prove to myself that I could still do it, that my disease wasn't taking away my favorite things. Then when that reason wasn't enough any longer, I pushed myself because I'd already paid for it - I didn't want to waste it.

Then came the point where we began working on our piece for the show at the end of the year. Once we began that, I needed to keep going. I had a part in the piece and if I wasn't there it would negatively affect the group. One time, during the warm-up/technique portion of class, I had to step out and sit down on the cold floor in the back hall because I was still experiencing the vertigo from my allergic reaction to an injection a few days earlier. But I made sure I came back to class before we began rehearsing our piece that night so that I wouldn't miss any new choreography, even though I still felt horribly crummy!

And then there was the issue of not being allowed to wear contacts. The ophthalmologist told me about 3/4 the way through the dance season that I could no longer wear them. I couldn't dance with my glasses on - they flew off every time I turned, or moved my head much at all. But I can't see enough without them to be able to learn new choreography, have very good balance or to feel comfortable dancing.

In the end, I was very proud of myself (I did, however, cheat and wear my contacts for the performance, after which my eyes felt horrible from wearing them!). The chance to perform again in front of an audience (including my family - and especially my daughter that shares my love of dance) was wonderful.

But even this experience caused issues in other areas of my life beyond the physical. There were times that I was questioned about why I couldn't do something because I was "too tired" but yet I could go to dance. I would try to explain my reasons for still going to dance - that I paid for it, or that I was a part of a group that was working together on a piece for the show – but it didn't always work in justifying why I could make it to dance but not do something else. I felt guilty about taking time away from my family's busy schedule each week to go to class. My guilt was increased by the fact that it was making others (and myself!) question why I could do that, but not other things.

It's not just the "physical" interests and hobbies that are being affected. I love photography - a life-style, semi-journalistic style of photography that captures the everyday moments and details of life. However using the mouse on the computer to edit the images is painful. The motor control issues also makes me more clumsy in these efforts. Each time I work on my images I'm reminded of this, and often have to stop simply because I can't use the mouse as well, or for as long. The fatigue and brain fog also mean that it's harder to convince myself to go work on them, and that when I do find the time and energy I'm far less efficient than I use to be.

So now, with these realizations of how I can no longer maintain my interests and hobbies, my questions become: When I can only keep small pieces of who I am, which ones do I keep? Which pieces and parts do I let go? When I have a more severely limited amount of energy, how do I balance what I have to and need to do for others with keeping the small piece of my former self that I need to hang on to in order to feel like myself, to continue to have hope that my "new normal" can still maintain a piece of my "old normal"? If I let all the "frivolous" things go in order to maintain the "necessities," how long until I'm unable to be happy and fulfilled enough to be myself? How do I decide what I can't or won't do in other areas of my life, or for other people, in order to have enough of myself to maintain something that I love?

Self-Concept

As I've said before, I'm a pleaser. I want people to like me. I want to make others happy. Some of my mental and emotional struggles with this disease come from my fear of what others will think about the way I'm acting or how others will view my ability (or lack of ability) to cope.

I can often cope with these external judgment issues by knowing that the people in my life that love me unconditionally will continue to do so, no matter how I'm coping with what's going on. And if others don't understand what I'm going through (or attempt to understand, as I'm not sure anyone can totally understand without experiencing it themselves), then that's on them and not on me. There's nothing I can do about how they react. All easier said than done, but sometimes it does help me deal with my issues of how others will view me.

However, much of my mental and emotional struggles come from my own self-concept. How I view myself. How I judge how I'm living up to my own expectations for myself. These struggles are far, far harder to brush off than the ones stemming from how others view me.

I've had tough times before. I've had times where one part of my life wasn't going spectacularly. Times when maybe I wasn't doing my absolute best at my job but I was a new mother and was putting my efforts there. Or when I was going through a divorce but was graduating with a PhD and moving into a different phase of my career.

We each have many ways that we define ourselves - I'm a mother, wife, daughter, sister, friend, educator, writer, speaker, photographer and dancer. I have always been smart, successful, industrious, efficient, caring, supportive, generous with my time and willing to do anything I could to help someone out.

While coping with this disease and all the many ways that it reaches into my life, I feel like I'm doing poorly in each and every part of the ways in which I define myself. Brian fog, pain, fatigue, fine motor control, stress and frustration are reaching into every single aspect of my life and causing havoc. I'm not being the best mother I can be. I'm not the wife I want to be for my husband. I'm not participating in friend and family relationships in the way that I'd like. I'm not working towards my career goals. I'm not enjoying hobbies and creative outlets. I'm not feeling very smart, successful, industrious or efficient. I'm not reaching out in caring, supportive ways, volunteering or supporting others as I would like.

Always before I could say "even though this one part of my life is struggling or not going so well right now, I have these other parts that I can be proud of and use to carry me through." It was OK that one part of my self-concept wasn't doing so well because I had other parts that were. But there's literally not a single aspect of my life that is not being affected by this disease.

Sometimes I feel useless. I feel like a failure. I feel like I have no redeeming qualities left to carry me through. Nothing to hold up to myself and be proud of, feel good about.

I know in my head that this isn't true, but I still feel that way sometimes.

As Others See Me

I'm concerned about how this disease affects how I see myself, my self-concept, but also how others see me. Despite my sharing of my innermost thoughts, concerns, complaints, etc., in this book and my blog, I do hide it on a daily basis. And apparently I hide it well.

A friend, that also happens to be my hair stylist for the past 8 years, read a draft of this book as a favor to me. When I walked into my appointment with her after she'd finished reading it she said she'd had no idea – that despite seeing me every 5 weeks for the past 8 years, during which I've struggled with this disease for at least the last 6 years.

We talked about the dubious nature of this ability to hide it. Should I be so good and consistent about hiding it? It leads to a lot of stress and anxiety on my part – such as when I struggle to keep up with others, to fulfill my obligations or when I feel like I'm letting people in my life down. And it also leads to misunderstandings – when others don't understand why I can't do things, why I'm tired, etc.

But if I don't hide it what do I become? A walking "sick person" that is constantly reminding others that I'm struggling with this disease? I don't want that – and I know nobody wants to be around that.

So where's the balance? Where's the magic amount of hiding it so as not to become my disease and completely lose myself and my interactions with others, but not to hide it so much that it's not fair to myself and my struggles? This is not an easy thing at all – and adds one more layer of things that I have to deal with as a sufferer of chronic, invisible disease. It truly affects all parts of my life.

I do worry about how others see me – I don't want people to judge me for not being able to volunteer or clean or pull my weight in any number of ways. My therapist keeps asking me who I'm worried about judging? Who is it that I'm concerned about? Those closest to me (family and closest friends) understand and love me no matter what. Those that don't understand, why am I letting their reactions and feelings affect me?

Again, it's about finding balance. I don't want to be narcissistic and only worry about me and how things affect me and not how I affect others. I want to be caring, compassionate, helpful – all the things that I feel like I've been in my life. I'm a pleaser – I want to be liked and respected. So where's the balance in caring about others and their needs but not letting the judgment of ignorant people (people that truly don't understand what it's like to live with these struggles) affect me? I don't know.

And tied into this struggle to balance how I let others' feelings about me affect me is the struggle to know when to tell someone what's going on with me. Does the random person that I don't really know but that doesn't understand why I say no to every volunteer request need to know why? I often feel the need to justify my "no" responses with why. I know everyone is busy and everyone has struggles but if everyone said "no" to everything then nothing would get done – volunteers are needed. But I simply can't do what I once could and I feel horrible saying no all the time. I often feel the need to justify myself when I say no. But I also don't want to hang my disease out there like for everyone. I don't mind sharing and educating, but is it everyone in the world's business why I say no to something? How do I decide which people need to know and which don't?

And if I do tell someone what's going on, when? At which point in a relationship do I try to explain what's going on with me and how it often affects my mood, my ability to volunteer, to follow through? When do I tell new friends the reason why I often need to cancel my plans with them or don't initiate plans because I never know when I'm going to have a "fatigue day" and not be able to do it?

All of these struggles may not seem like big things, but when you put them all together and you add it in with the struggles for diagnosis, effective treatment, medical professionals that fit with you, not to mention the physical effects of the disease, it's all very hard.

Work

My current job has been the biggest blessing I could have asked for. It has allowed me to work from home several days a week and given me flexibility that I would not have had in my previous life as a high school teachers. I could freely schedule doctor appointments, rest when I needed it, work when I felt best and not feel the added pressure of being "on" in a workplace environment when I felt so poorly.

But my current position is a grant-funded position that I knew would end when I took it. There is 15 months left of the grant, but it's definitely time to start seriously looking for the next step.

Am I even going to be capable of doing another job? I have said many times over the past few years that I could not have been a full-time high school teacher (as I was the first 10 years of my career) with all that I've had going on recently. I physically could not have done it. Not with the spells of extreme fatigue, the pain, the nasty reactions to medications, the doctor appointments, and so on. When this all went into full swing, I felt like by the time my current position ended it would all be under control. I'd be back to somewhat closer to normal. I knew I'd never be cured of this disease, but I thought that surely in the 4.5 years that I then had left of my job, I'd be able to get it under control enough to be able to function in a more traditional environment.

Here I am, years later, with the end of my highly flexible, position looming and I'm no closer to having this disease managed. In fact, I'm even worse than I was before...in both number of symptoms and severity.

I had an all-day interview for a university faculty position. It involved 4 or 5 meetings with various people, lunch and teaching a class for college students studying to be teachers about using educational technology to "get outside the classroom".

I really liked the people, the place, the energy and just about everything about it. I felt more like myself that day than I have in a long time. I had interesting discussions on educational technology and teacher preparation. I chatted with many very nice people, and in general felt like myself.

And then by the time I got home, I crashed. It took me about two days to not feel absolutely and completely drained - just back to my "normal level" of tired and painful. Clearly that "feeling like my old self" is not sustainable. I can do it for short periods - but there's no way I could do it day in and day out.

Will I even be able to do something else? I have to. I have no choice. I have to help support my family. Will I physically be able to handle it? What if helping to support my family each day means that I come home and immediately climb into bed (which is what I did after that all-day interview)? Will helping to support my family mean anything if then I don't have the energy and ability to spend time with them and be the mom and wife I want and need to be? I already have issues with feeling like I'm failing at both of those parts of my life and that's without the daily drain of working in a more traditional environment.

And there's even more to be concerned about than the physical ability to work a full-time job. Brain fog is seriously in the way! I've heard many people talk about the "impostor syndrome" throughout my life. It's a phenomenon that happens with highly educated or esteemed people when they doubt that they really know as much as their accolades lead others to believe. Many are afraid that someday others will figure out that they're not as smart as the others first thought - that they're an "impostor."

Brain fog takes impostor syndrome to a whole new level! Not only do I have the normal impostor syndrome feeling of "someone will figure out that I'm not as smart as a PhD is supposed to be," but now I have "Brain fog is causing me to not even be as smart as I was when I was mildly worried I'd be called an impostor!"

I also don't want to try another job and fail. As you saw in the chapter on my self-concept, I'm already feeling like all the various aspects of my life are a mess. I already sometimes feel like a failure. To confirm it by trying to work full time and not being able to is a frightening thought. It's one thing to feel like a possible failure - it's quite another thing to be proven correct. I know that illness making me incapable of doing something isn't the same things as "being a failure" - but once again, just because I know something isn't true doesn't mean that I stop feeling the feelings.

Not only do I worry that others I work with will think (or confirm) that I'm an impostor, but I worry that I won't be dependable for them. I've always been a person that would volunteer to do something and then get it done. Now, I can't even remember things - let alone be depended upon to get them done on time and like they should be done. I don't want to let others down at work any more than I want to let my family down. Will I be able to pull my own weight or will I be the one that no one wants to work with because I can't be relied upon?

There is also the very real issue of lost time due to doctor's appointments. In the last 6 weeks I've had a doctor's appointment, procedure or test at least 1 time per week. Each is at the teaching hospital an hour away. Both the rheumatologist and neurologist kept me waiting for almost an hour past my appointment time before they came into the room, adding to the total time burden. Each of those appointments would have meant a day off work if I didn't have this flexible job schedule. That's 20% loss work time over the last 6 weeks.

The concern for lost or diminished ability to work (due to the disease itself as well as the frequent medical appointments) is a real one - and one that could very quickly impact my family. Two independent studies showed that the annual indirect cost of Sjögren's was between $12,150 (lower range) and $21,369 (higher range). This indirect costs figure included "all non-medical costs due to autoimmune disease, including time lost from current work (lower range) and time lost from inability to work at all or to work full-time (higher range). Indirect costs also include the cost of hiring help for tasks that the patients cannot do due to their illness."*

Autoimmune disease is the fourth leading cause of dis-

---

*   http://www.diabetesed.net/page/_files/autoimmune-diseases.pdf

ability for women in the US†. Between the physical concerns of moving on to another job and the psychological concerns of not being able to be what I once was - there is a great deal of stress in my life concerning my career and where exactly it's headed.

† http://www.aarda.org/autoimmune-information/autoimmune-disease-in-women/

Friendships

My chronic illness has definitely had an impact on my relationships with friends in the last few years. I built up friendships after my divorce. I spent more time with friends, I found people that I enjoyed hanging out with. I had fun with them. Most of them became family friends - either our children were friends and the adults became friends or the adults were friends and our children began to play together as well. But unfortunately most of that has stopped in the last few years.

It takes energy to be social, especially when you're not really "feeling it." I don't want to be a "Debbie downer" all the time. I know my true friends understand that I'm struggling but that doesn't mean they want to be around someone that is always in a funk. And I don't want to be the person in the group that acts that way.

I don't make plans because I don't know if I'll be too tired or hurting to go through with them. I avoid situations with lots of people because the more people there are the more I have to put on a happy face and chit-chat. And I often want to leave early from things because I just get worn out. And then I end up exactly like I described in the "isolation" chapter - turning down offers often enough that then people stop extending them or just simply don't think to include me because I haven't been around lately.

Sometimes it's good to be able to "escape" for a while
and be in casual social situations. It feels good to pretend to
be normal. However, I'm always aware that I can't sustain it
for long. I'm always aware that it means less energy I'll have
for my family or other things that need to get done at home or
work. It's another example of having to choose. Yes, all people
are choosing to use part of their available time and energy with
their friendships, but my time and energy pool is much smaller
to begin with. There's more guilt associated with even taking
a small portion of energy and spending it with friends rather
than on necessary activities.

It's easier to be around a small group, and of people that
know me well. They know that I'm struggling and not myself
and I feel more comfortable that they aren't judging me. I do
worry a lot about what others are thinking. I don't volunteer at
the kids' school or in their activities like I used to do. I'm not
as outgoing as I once was. I don't join in and chat with others
like I used to do. I worry that others will think I'm stuck up,
not pulling my weight, exaggerating my symptoms or using my
illness as an excuse.

At what point do I explain myself? My friends are
aware that I have an autoimmune disease. But when do I explain it to people that don't know? For example, do I explain
it to my kids' teachers each year so that they know why I don't
volunteer? It feels like making excuses or sharing too much
information to explain it, but then I feel as if people will get the
wrong idea about me if I don't.

It all reminds me of those memes that travel around
on social media that remind us to not judge others because we

never know what their personal struggles are. We don't know what's going on in the life of the waitress that's distracted or the traveler that seems rude rushing through lines. I like to think I've always been a compassionate person - I think it's in the nature of most educators to be that way. But these struggles have brought it even more into focus. I don't want or need to share my struggles with everyone that I encounter, yet I also don't want them judging me without knowing what my struggles are.

Even the most common of social scenarios takes on a new light for me. The greeting of "Hi, how are you?" that is spoken hundreds of times a day makes me stop and pause. The automatic reflex is to answer "Great. How are you?" But then I stop and think "I'm not really great. Why do I say that?" It's used as a greeting in our culture rather than a true question so often that it's become automatic.

There are times when a friend truly is stopping and asking me how I'm doing - not just the greeting, but truly asking the question. I'm grateful for those moments because I can tell they're concerned and they're trying to check on me. However, the best I can usually get out is "eh, alright," because if I go into any more detail than that I'll tear up and likely not be able to get out much at all. And even if the person is genuinely interested in how I'm doing and stopping to listen to my response rather than using it as an expanded version of "Hi"as we so often do, I'm pretty sure they're not ready for the full emotional flood that would be coming their way if I fully answered their question.

I do appreciate when someone sincerely asks how I'm doing. I also greatly appreciate random messages of "I'm thinking of you" or "You're in my prayers." I think most people just don't know what to say. We want to say something when someone else is struggling, but we often don't know what to say. So we say things like "Hope you feel better soon!" I know people are well meaning, but I'm not going to get better soon - it's not a cold or flu that I'll suffer through and then move on as normal.

My struggle to remain social and maintain friendships is just one more area of my life that this disease has reached. There truly is nothing safe from it and that fact feels crushing to me.

Marriage

Autoimmune disease has also had an impact on my relationship with my husband. Just as it has affected my friendships in many different ways, it also affects my marriage in several ways.

I've already talked about how much we depend on him for our family's day-to-day functioning and it's been a big change. In the beginning, we split household duties pretty evenly - we both like to cook and we split up cleaning chores. Now it's pretty much him doing it all. I've been the one in a family to do it all before and it's not fun - I don't want him to have to feel that way.

I am not the same woman I was when we fell in love. I'm much more distant, reserved and quiet. I'm less affectionate and not up for fun things like I used to be. I know that I'm not acting like myself and I don't like it, but yet that's what I can manage right now. It's not fair to him - none of it.

It took a long time for me to convince him that it wasn't about him or our relationship. I can completely understand why he would think that was the case - if someone began to withdrawal and become distant with me I'd be afraid it was personal as well. But it's not. It has no reflection on how I feel about him. If I could share what's going on with anyone in my life, it would be him. I just have such a hard time. I have a hard time admitting all of these faults and issues. But I also have a hard time literally getting it out. Each time I try to start to talk about any of these issues I've written about, I immediately begin to tear up and get chocked up and can't talk about it.

It's also been hard for him to see me "put on a happy face" and act normal around other people and then turn around and come home only to revert back to my "shell." He wonders why I can be social around other people but then come home and go back to withdrawn. The best I can explain it is that I pretend to be fine around other people because I feel like I need to - but that with him I feel like I can be how I truly feel. It feels safe to let the false front down around him. I also can't maintain the false "normal-ness" for extended periods of time, and after I've done it around other people I'm often tired and worn out and just want to lay down and be alone. Again, it's not fair to him. To see glimpses of the "old me" when we're around other people, only to come home with the quiet, tired, hurting me.

I want to be myself again - I really do. But between the physical pain and fatigue and all the mental and emotional stresses and worries, I just can't sustain it.

My greatest fear is that he'll get tired of it. He'll realize that this is unfair for him and that he doesn't have to live like this. Just the thought is terrifying to me, but I also would understand it - after all, even when I had just a hint of how difficult this was all going to be when I first received an autoimmune diagnosis, I asked him if he was sure he wanted to still marry me. Again, no one knows what life is going to hand them - we all might end up dealing with things that we had no idea were headed our way and feel like we "didn't sign up for it."

But it's different knowing you *might* have to deal with a loved ones' chronic illness and knowing that you *definitely* will have to deal with it for many, many years.

My writing has helped. It's given me an outlet that I can use to express how I feel and what I'm dealing with and it's given him a way to see those thoughts, feelings and struggles. It's not the most conventional of ways to communicate, but it's the way I can get it out and he can read it. It's helped me feel better, knowing that I am communicating with him. I feel better knowing that I'm expressing myself and letting him in, even if I'm only able to do it through writing. It's helped him understand what it is that I'm dealing with, be more patient with me and be better able to understand my moods and what's going on that might cause me to have better days or worse days. I've noticed him ask more questions about my doctor's appointment and what's going on with me, even researching my disease himself. I know it doesn't make up for everything he's having to deal with as I deal with this disease, but it helps relieve a little bit of stress from me knowing that I'm at least able to communicate in some way.

As a side note – when reading through the book for last edits and changes, this was the only chapter that made me cry. I'm so numb to all of this sometimes that I don't cry when I read it (and I'm trying to read it as a proofreader and not someone emotionally attached to it). Although I probably feel more guilt about feeling like I let my children down than over the way I feel like I let my husband down, the kids are stuck with me, they're not going anywhere at least until they're grown. But my husband is here by choice and I'm so thankful that he choices it – I think that's why this chapter hits me so hard.

When Naps are No Fun

When I had small children, I never understood why they fought nap time. I always thought to myself "If someone would tell me to take a nap everyday, I'd love it...I'd never fight it!" Of course, this was from the perspective of a normal, healthy, energetic, busy, efficient, successful mother of two young children.

Several years later, I'm a far cry from that person. I've described how I have to cut things out of my life - and choose between things that I shouldn't have to choose between - in order to have enough energy to function throughout a day. I've talked about the realities of trying to maintain a successful career with autoimmune disease.

But I haven't talked about my naps. I feel like it's a dirty little secret. I feel like if I told people how often I take naps they would all look at me with either envy or judgment.

Envy would be from those busy mothers of young children that would love the time to take a leisurely nap in the afternoon. But really, I don't think it's the nap per-say (at least as long as you're getting a full night sleep - which I was as that was at the point since my kids both slept through the night and allowed me a full 8 hours of sleep at night) that most would be jealous of. It's more the idea that you have "free time" in which you could choose to take a nap. Guilt-free ability to use time in any way you wish - and if that way happens to be a nap, then so be it. I think that's what I was wishing for when thinking I'd love to have mandated nap time each day as I watched my toddlers fight it - the block of time when I had no other require-ments...just time to "waste" and have zero guilt or shame associ-ated with it.

Judgment would be from everyone else that is tired, too, but keeps on going throughout their day and makes it to the end without taking a nap, during which their other duties are being shirked. That judgment, coming from my own self, is what kept me from taking naps when my kids did in those early days of motherhood - I can't take a nap...I have laundry to do, a kitchen to clean, toys to put away before they wake up and drag them all out again, work to do, etc. What kind of mother, wife and graduate student/science education writer/"all the other career things I was working on" person would I be if I chose to take a nap over some of the other things I needed to get done?

My desire to take those naps all those years ago had more to do with the luxurious feeling of taking time for a leisurely nap and less to do with the actual fatigue of my body (again - this was once I got past late night feedings and other sleep-depriving moments of early motherhood).

I've always been a person that needed a full night sleep to feel good. I was never someone that could routinely function on little sleep. But now it's a whole new level of fatigue.

For example, I slept 9 hours last night (11pm - 8am). I then slept from 10:30am-12:30pm. That's 11 hours of sleep - almost half my day. That 10:30am nap was because I literally could not stay awake any longer. I was trying to work. I got to the point where my brain wasn't able to concentrate on the work that I needed to do. It was a physical fatigue that was definitely affecting my ability to concentrate and work.

The best way I can describe it to people is like the fatigue in early pregnancy. That feeling of your body is heavy and is pulling you down into sleep and you simply can't fight it any more. It's definitely not a "I think I'll go take a nap" moment because I'm bored, procrastinating, don't feel like doing any of the things I need to do or any other reason. It's a deep physical need to sleep.

It's hard to wake up. You'd think after 9 hours of sleep and 2 hours of napping that I'd wake up refreshed. Wrong. It's like dragging myself up from deep underwater with cement blocks tied to my feet. I have to will myself to wake up and get up. I probably could have slept for another 3 hours but I simply have to get something done today.

When I took naps for other reasons (boredom, leisure, procrastination, etc.) in years past, I wouldn't be able to fall asleep that night. My body had slept the previous night, and during the nap the day and I simply wasn't tired when I went to bed that night. Then I'd want a nap the next day because I hadn't slept well that night and I'd make myself fight through it to get back on a regular night-time sleeping pattern. That's simply not the case now. I'll fall asleep tonight and sleep another 9 hours without any problem at all - despite the 11 hours of sleep I got last night and today.

I can fight it for the short term. I can go a couple of days without napping if I simply have to - if work, or doctor's appointments, or kids' activities simply requires it and there's no way to meet these minimum requirements of my daily life while addressing the fatigue when it hits each day. But I can't sustain that long. My body will pay for those days of pushing through.

This is why I often have to choose between things, why I'm having to give things up, why I have immense guilt at not being the best wife, mother, friend, worker, etc., as I know I could, should and want to be - because I have such a deep, physical fatigue that I just can't ignore.

If you compare the 8-hour per day sleep that is recommended with my 11 hour sleep last night/today, over the course of a year that's an extra 1095 hours of sleep I'll be getting. That's 45.6 days. Do you have any idea what I could do with those 45 days if I could get them back? I have goals. I have careers ideas and plans. I have the desire to clean my house. I want to have energy and time to play with my kids and hang out with my husband. I'd do just about anything to have those 45 days back this year.

So, please don't ever say to someone struggling with chronic fatigue things like "I wish I could lay around and rest or take naps every day" or "Must be nice to take that time for yourself each day" or "My day makes me tired, too, but I have too much to do with my family/work/etc. to take time out."

Because, trust me, the daily naps aren't fun. They're riddled with self-imposed guilt and judgment, as well as the fear of external judgment. They are filled with heartache at what I know I'm missing because of them. They force me to give up things that I love, want and need to do. If I could have my busy, hectic, non-stop life back, I would give up these daily naps in a heartbeat. They are not leisurely, luxurious or pleasurable. They are not fun.

Asking for Help

"Just let me know if I can do anything!"

That's such a kind offer and I've received it a few times over the last few years. I always answer it with "I will!"

Only I never do.

Not because I don't appreciate the offer. Not because I don't need help. Not because I don't think they mean it. So if it's not for all these reasons, then why don't I ever take anyone up on their offer?

For one, I'm so overwhelmed that I don't even know where to start asking for help. There are so many aspects that are causing struggle that I'm not sure what to address first.

Second, because the things I need help with are things that I'm supposed to be able to do myself. Run my kids around, clean the house, do laundry, cook meals. These are things that aren't that difficult. It's not like I'm moving to a different house or putting in a privacy fence - both of those things I had no problem asking for help (just ask my dad, I'm always asking for his help with those kinds of things). I have no problem asking for help for big, infrequent projects or tasks. It's the little, day-to-day things that are hard to ask for help with.

I have enough guilt that my husband is picking up so much slack for me around the house - if I actually called someone and asked them to come over and clean the kitchen for me, I would be unbelievably embarrassed! I mean it's not like I have a broken leg or am recovering from surgery! How in the world could I lay around and "rest" from "fatigue" while someone else cleans my house? Or how can I accept meals from someone in front of my children when, on the outside, there's nothing wrong with their mom! There's simply no way I could do that! I'd feel so spoiled, selfish and wrong doing such things!

And this exactly exemplifies the fight that I have going on within myself. On the one hand I struggle to explain to people just how serious this condition is - despite it's invisibility and the way that it seems like just an exaggeration of what everyone with a busy life experiences as they age. I've spent much of this book describing all the different, very real ways that it impacts every aspect of my life. And every bit of it has been true and non-exaggerated.

But then I turn around and say "It's not like I have a broken leg or am recovering from surgery!" It's the same issue I have with giving a pain rating on the "no pain to the worst pain you can imagine" pain scale. Surely what I'm going through isn't bad enough to have someone come over and clean the kitchen for me. Surely I don't need someone to cook meals for my family. Yet I didn't think twice about accepting it when my mom cleaned the apartment for me after I had knee surgery in college. And I gave a very sincere "thank you" without a hint of guilt when two friends fixed meals for us while I was recovering from thyroid surgery years ago.

Not only am I in the middle of fighting to convince

others that this disease is real and impact-ful, but I'm fighting to convince myself as well. I'm still trying to come to grips with the fact that I may need help and accommodations to get through life.

It's also a matter of pride and independence. I've always been able to take care of myself and do things. When my husband asked if I wanted him to put in the screws on the treadmill as we were putting it together last year, I was determined to prove to myself that I could still do such a simple task. It made my hands hurt even worse, probably took way longer than it should, and definitely put me in a worse mood than was necessary...but I was determined to still be able to do things I've done in the past. I simply have a hard time admitting that I need help or that I can't do everything by myself.

How can I ask for help when I need help with nothing (because all the little tasks are just that - little tasks) yet I need help with everything.

Accommodations

Accommodations are ways to change tasks, do things differently or use other tools to ease a task. It is possible to make accommodations for various difficulties as they come up. Some are easier to implement than others. Some are more readily available. Some require creativity and persistence to develop.

Great resources for finding accommodations are discussion boards of people with similar diseases or struggles – asking what others have figured out to do in similar situations. A good source for work-related accommodations is the Job Accommodations Network (www.askjan.org) - it has great American Disabilities Act information and can be searched by disease or symptoms.

The problem is that, just like these diseases and their symptoms, one size doesn't fit all. Just because you have a specific disease doesn't mean you have the same struggles and roadblocks and it doesn't mean the same accommodations work for you. Every person is unique and every situation is unique.

And to added to the challenge is the fact that what each person needs is likely a moving target. What works for now may not work later. What you can do fine or reasonably well today may not be possible in a few months. You can often feel like you're running to constantly stay ahead and find ways to do things that you used to do.

Sometimes it's a matter of getting a different tool. For example, at work the regular PC keyboards increase my pain when typing. I asked for a scissor type keyboard – the keys are flatter (more like a laptop keyboard) and require less force and distance to press them down. I asked for a trackpad instead of a mouse because scrolling and clicking on a traditional mouse was increasing pain.

Sometimes it's changing the way you do something. For example, hanging clothes is easier than folding them for me so I hang my pants rather than fold them.

Sometimes it's changing when you do something – if you have times of the day when pain or fatigue is worse, rearrange your schedule. This doesn't work for me as I have random fatigue and pain – I never know when it's going to strike so I can't plan around it. I could wake up and know it's going to be a bad day or I could be relatively OK in the morning to feel like I've been hit by a truck by afternoon.

I've found the real challenge is in accommodating for fatigue. It's easier to find a way to work around a physical challenge than fatigue. I can use different tools, software, technology, etc., to get my work done easier with my pain. However, the only accommodation for fatigue is rest. But then how do you get everything done? We still have the same amount of time each day, but our bodies demand rest more than others. I still have the same demands of personal care, family life, parenting, social needs, etc., that everyone else does. But I have limited time because of the rest periods needed for fatigue. So even if you can have a flexible schedule to get your work done during your "better" times, you still have less time than the rest of the world. You still have to figure out how to get everything done in less time – being careful not to push too hard or you'll face a backlash of increased fatigue.

You often hear people say "we all have the same amount of time in the day" or "'I didn't have time' isn't an excuse – you just chose to do other things with your time." But, no, I truly don't have the same amount of time as everyone else. My body does not physically allow me to use the same amount of time that other people are able to use. That logic simply doesn't work with someone struggling with a fatigue-causing disease. (Oh, and don't forget to add in all the many, many doctor's appointments and tests that take up our time as well!)

Waiting for the Finish

This book was almost done after 3 months of writing. Yet, here I am over a year after beginning it, just now finishing it. Why the delay?

Yes, fatigue, pain and the demands of everyday life are a part of the reason – it's hard to fit in time for writing when you have other things to do with that precious time during the day and it's hard to type 50,000 words when your hands hurt. But that's only a small part of it. My desire to get this story out there – both for myself and for others – was great enough to overcome those challenges for the short amount of time it would've taken to finish the last couple of chapters. After all, it only took a few hours when I did decide to sit down and finish it – I could have done it in the last 9 months.

The real reason I didn't finish it for so long was because I was waiting for it to "wrap up." I was waiting for the climax – for me to begin a new treatment and for it to have some benefit and for me to be able to say to myself and my readers "see, if you just push through and self-advocate enough then you'll reach a point where things are stable and acceptable, if not great or what they once were." It took me several months to even figure out that was the reason I'd stopped writing – I hadn't even articulated to myself that this was what was going on.

As much as I've talked in this book about how it's chronic, life-long, there's no cure, it affects every part of your life, etc., I still had this strange, extremely illogical, feeling that there would be a wrap-up moment. A moment when I could complete the story arch – girl gets sick, girl struggles with un-diagnosis, mis-diagnosis, bad doctors, and comes through to find an acceptable equilibrium in life and is now sharing pearls of wisdom for how you can get through it, too. After all, that's how other books I've read on these types of things happen. Everyone wraps up the book with their Zen-like advice on how to make peace with your disease, how to keep hope, how to not let it define you and so on.

But that's just the point with these diseases – there is no "culminating moment" when everything is wrapped up. Yes, I can tell myself all those pieces of advice about not letting it define me, and yes I can work each day to live in that way. But there is no final moment in this journey. There will always be new symptoms, worsening symptoms, tests for other autoimmune diseases overlapping my current diagnosis, etc. There will also be struggles with physical limitations and the realities of this disease.

It's absolutely mind-boggling to me that I had to have a "realization moment" of this even after the years of struggling with it – that I wasn't aware of it all along or at least much sooner than I was. I think it had been a vague, fuzzy idea in the back of my mind somewhere, but it was a little shocking to me when it crystalized into a cohesive though of "I can't wait for this story to wrap up before finishing the writing – it's not going to wrap up."

It's been a year since I started writing and I'm not there

yet. It's been 6 months since I fired Dr. C with the letter after my last disappointing appointment with him. I have an appointment next month 1200 miles from home with one of the top Sjögren's specialists in the country. I made the appointment a week after writing the letter to Dr. C. It's a 7-month wait to get into to see this next doctor (I guess he'd be "Dr. D" – maybe it's a sign that I'm "Dr. Dempewolf" – maybe the "Dr. D" thing will be good luck!).

I have a sense of cautious hope. I hope that he will take my symptoms, all my symptoms, seriously. I don't think he'll be able to fix it all – after all there is no cure for this disease. But I just want him to take all my symptoms seriously – to really listen and respond in a way that I feel heard and understood. But at this point in my journey I'm definitely cautious. I've felt the devastation of having my hopes crash and don't want to set myself up for that again.

And I don't want to wait until that appointment is over to finish this book – what if it's a many-month-long process and I'm still no closer (like I experienced with Dr. C)? I have no doubt that it will take more than this upcoming appointment to get things to even a semi "wrapped-up" point. At some point I have to finish and put it out there and continue to update on happenings through the blog, www.asmybodyattacksitself.com.

The Wrap-Up

Despite my description of my "realization" that there is no "wrapping up" point in this story – no neat little ending where we see how the journey concludes and can learn lessons from it, I have learned a few things up to this point worth sharing in a final chapter.

First, keep track of things. Keep journals – either actual paper journals or electronic journals through one of the many, many available technology tools and apps for journaling. This helps with the symptom creep. Keeping track of what you do and how you feel can help you see patterns as well as symptom creep that might otherwise not become apparent as you continually adjust to a "new normal." I've tried several various apps to help me do this and none of them have exactly the features I need to easily keep all the information that I'd like to keep – the irony is that I can code and have created apps and could create one for myself to journal the way that I'd like to…but that dang fatigue prevents me from being able to do so!

Second, writing is a wonderful way of processing. Whether it's a part of those journals or whether it's a blog or other public means of sharing information, writing can often help people organize their thoughts. It doesn't have to be public – you can even create a blog that is private and only for you.

You don't have to worry about your writing not being good enough for others to read or it being something any one would be interested in reading. Do it for yourself. I've written a lot – this is my 4th book, I've published a dozen research articles and blog posts for both my medical issues and science education, and I've taught a lot of high school students. Writing is a wonderful way to get your thoughts out of the vague, fuzzy stage and clear them up for your own understanding. Don't worry about it being fuzzy when you start – use the writing process to clear them up. People often think they have to think through everything and have a plan before they begin writing – but that just means they likely never start writing because they're never clear on it all. Just start and see where it gets you.

Third, research is important but be careful of falling down that rabbit hole. These diseases are as unique as the people suffering from them. Although I hear my experiences echoed by those that share their experiences and there are common aspects (the difficulty in getting a diagnosis, the ebb and flow of symptoms, the difficulties associated with invisible and chronic illnesses, etc.), the details of each story may be different. Test results may be different. Symptom onset may not be in the same order or intensity. Different people respond to medications differently and so on. And there's so much overlap in diseases that you can often think you have all of the 80+ auto-immune diseases because you have a little piece of each one. So use your internet time wisely – judge the source of the information carefully and don't rely on or discount any information because it doesn't exactly match your experience – these things are immensely complicated and personal!

And the last lesson I've learned is to advocate. But there are two parts to it – to advocate for yourself with others and to advocate for yourself *to* yourself.

When advocating for yourself to others, keep these things in mind:

- Never forget that you have the right to step back and look at the information with a fresh eye and perhaps re-diagnose. You always have the right to seek another opinion or to look for other care providers.
- Ask for those letters from specialists to primary care doctors be sent to you as well. They won't always do it (I asked for it at KU med and received copies of only 3 letters out of the dozen or more appointments I had).
- You have the right to request copies of your medical records. They may charge a fee for processing, printing and mailing them, but you do have the right to see ALL of your records – including those letters sent to your primary care doctor.
- Don't feel like a "bother" when contacting a doctor. I often felt like I was a bother when contacting them to follow up with a prescription that hadn't been approved yet, with side-effects that I felt were important or when new symptoms appear. We are paying them to deal with these things. It is their job and their business. If they treat you like a bother then you need to look for another care provider.
- Doctors get tunnel vision (like when Dr. C was "stuck" on describing it as numbness and tingling no matter how many times I told him that wasn't what was going on). You may need to tell them "listen, you're stuck on this idea and that's not it. Can you please take a look with an open mind or listen with a fresh set of ears."
- Doctors and nurses can sometimes get appointments for you with other doctors quicker than you can (I called Dr. C and he got me into the neurologist quicker than when I'd called the neurologist and complained about

worsening symptoms myself).

When advocating for myself *to* myself, these are the things I constantly need to be reminded of:

- Change your expectations for yourself. You cannot do what you once did. You must reset your baseline explanations. Be realistic. Unrealistic expectations don't do anyone any good.
- When worrying about what others think of you – if they are people that you should worry about then talk to them and if necessary educate them. If they are not people that you should be worrying about their judgments then you have to let it go.
- You didn't ask for this disease. It's not your fault.
- You do the best you can when you can.
- You're coping the best you can for the circumstances you're in.
- It is real. It is true. You're not imagining it. You're not lazy. You're not attention seeking. You're not exaggerating (If I was making stuff up, it wouldn't be this – my life was so much better before it that I wouldn't actively choose this!)
- Don't "fake it" too much – don't put on a happy face too much – it can cause you to fail to validate your feelings and cause unrealistic expectations in others.
- You will never be "over it." Just like the disease has no cure – the grief process is continuous and has no cure. You will like have moments of grief over the "lost" aspects of your life from time to time – there will never be a moment where from the time it all begins that you are completely at peace with this and are "over it." But there will also be times when you are as OK as possible with your "new normal."

These things are not easy – they are not things I've mastered, or am even very good at. But they are things that I know will help me as a part of my inner dialog. They are things that I know are true logically even if I have a hard time with their "truth" emotionally. It's a choice each day to believe them – both logically and emotionally – and hopefully writing them down will help others as well as myself!

Acknowledgements

I want to thank Jenny Conner for reading the draft of this book for me - and for telling me that everyone I know should read this when she was done!

Thank you to Lynn Wagner Knight for encouraging me to write and share my thoughts for others to read.

Thank you to all the online fellow autoimmune disease people that have given me such great feedback on the sharing of my struggles.

Thank you to my friends and family that have put up with mood swings, pain, tears, frustration, anger and all the other things I've gone through in dealing with this disease over the years!

And most of all, I am immensely grateful for my children, Caleb and Shana, for being so fabulous and my husband, Kevin, for choosing to love us. Without you guys I wouldn't be who I am.

About the Author

I am a wife, mother of two amazing children, scientist, educator, photographer, dancer, author, speaker, creator of educational technology and many other things.

I was on track for a very successful career in science education. After 10 years of teaching high school chemistry, which included winning regional and national awards, being granted a National Board Certification, and authoring a nationally published high school chemistry textbook as well as many research articles, I received my PhD in education. I was poised to move into the next phase of my career - headed towards working with teachers. Whether that was in a university education department as a professor or working as an independent consultant, I was passionate about making a difference in the way science is taught in our schools.

Four years ago, however, I was diagnosed with an autoimmune disease. I have spent those years struggling to maintain pieces of myself, my goals and aspirations, and my roles as mother and wife all while battling chronic pain, fatigue, mis-diagnosis and medication after medication that provides no relief.

Although I've written three books and many articles in my career, I never imagined I'd write a book about a personal journey.

Yet here it is, and I can honestly say it's one of the things I'm most proud of in my life.